Telehealth: Strategies for Establishing Pharmacy Practice Models in Ambulatory Care Settings

CHRISTINA E. DEREMER, PharmD, BCPS, BCACP, FASHP

Clinical Associate Professor
Department of Pharmacotherapy and Translational Research
College of Pharmacy
University of Florida
Gainesville, Florida

ashp®

Any correspondence regarding this publication should be sent to the publisher, American Society of Health-System Pharmacists, 4500 East-West Highway, Suite 900, Bethesda, MD 20814, attention: Special Publishing.

Vice President, Publishing Office: Daniel J. Cobaugh, PharmD, DABAT, FAACT

Editorial Director, Special Publishing: Lori N. Justice, PharmD

Editorial Coordinator, Special Publishing: Elaine Jimenez

Director, Production and Platform Services, Publishing Operations: Johnna M. Hershey, BA

Cover Design: DeVall Advertising

Page Design: David Wade

Library of Congress Cataloging-in-Publication Data

Names: DeRemer, Christina E., editor. | American Society of Health-System Pharmacists, issuing body.
Title: Telehealth : strategies for establishing pharmacy practice models in ambulatory care settings / [edited by] Christina E. DeRemer.
Other titles: Telehealth (DeRemer)
Description: Bethesda, MD : American Society of Health-System Pharmacists, [2021] | Includes bibliographical references and index. | Summary: "Telehealth is a valuable tool for the profession of pharmacy to extend its reach to patients for the provision of medication management and complex patient care. Telehealth services have grown significantly over recent years and have been leveraged expressly during the COVID-19 global pandemic. These services have the potential to improve patient access to care, cost efficiencies, and quality while meeting consumer demand. This book, "Telehealth: strategies for establishing pharmacy telehealth practice models in ambulatory care settings," will serve as a guide to pharmacists who are beginning to implement telehealth services, and will also serve as a valuable resource to those with existing services by providing insight on best practices and revenue opportunities"—Provided by publisher.
Identifiers: LCCN 2021043113 (print) | LCCN 2021043114 (ebook) | ISBN 9781585286911 (paperback) | ISBN 9781585286928 (adobe pdf) | ISBN 9781585286935 (epub)
Subjects: MESH: Pharmaceutical Services | Telemedicine | Ambulatory Care
Classification: LCC RS122.2 (print) | LCC RS122.2 (ebook) | NLM QV 737.1 | DDC 362.17/820285—dc23
LC record available at https://lccn.loc.gov/2021043113
LC ebook record available at https://lccn.loc.gov/2021043114

ISBN: 978-1-58528-691-1 (paperback)

ISBN: 978-1-58528-692-8 (Adobe pdf)

ISBN: 978-1-58528-693-5 (ePub)

10 9 8 7 6 5 4 3 2 1

CONTENTS

DOI 10.37573/9781585286928.FM

PREFACE

"When we think of cheetahs, we think about their ability to go fast. What we don't often think about is their ability to change directions while going fast, or the way they get back up to speed once they've had to pivot to maintain performance."

John C Maxwell

During the COVID-19 pandemic, many healthcare "cheetahs" have been fighting this virus; both inside and outside the hospital. Due to the rapid pace for evolving strategies and information discoveries, healthcare professionals had to become adaptable and pivot practices quickly to not only target care to those affected by the virus but also simultaneously adjust management tactics and delegation of resources to maintain care for chronic, stable health needs. Despite the availability of telehealth as a care platform for years, the pandemic shifted its utility to a level never reached previously or even considered necessary. The capability for remote access served as a tool for the ambulatory pharmacy "cheetahs" to pivot and regain speed quickly.

An example: In a large, integrated healthcare system in Utah (Intermountain Healthcare), embedded ambulatory pharmacists were able to make the rapid shift to delivering care via telehealth during the early days of the COVID-19 pandemic. Their work helped bridge an important care gap while other healthcare professionals established telehealth processes. The smooth and quick transition to telehealth was facilitated by insightful preparation, value-based payment models, and professional flexibility of the pharmacists. The growth of pharmacist-delivered telehealth is filling an important need to simplify and increase patient access to care.

Christina E. DeRemer, Jeffery L Olson, and Angelina Vascimini

DOI 10.37573/9781585286928.FM

CONTRIBUTORS

Holly Causey Canupp, PharmD, BCACP, CPP, CDCES

Clinical Pharmacist Practitioner, Duke University Hospital
Duke University Hospital – Department of Pharmacy

Eric Dietrich, PharmD, BCACP, CPC-A, CPB, CEMC

Clinical Associate Professor
Department of Pharmacotherapy and Translational Research, University of Florida College of Pharmacy

Megan Dorrell, PharmD, BCACP

Clinical Director, Ambulatory Care Pharmacy
Community Health Network, Pharmacy Department

Heather Jones, PharmD, MS

Pharmacy Manager, Regional Oncology Services
Cleveland Clinic

Mary Ann Kliethermes, BS Pharm, PharmD, FAPhA, FCIOM

Director of Medication Safety and Quality
American Society of Health–System Pharmacists

Joe Lassiter, PharmD, MS

President and Chief Pharmacy Informatics Officer
The Robertson Group (TRG) LLC

Brody Maack, PharmD, BCACP, CTTS

Associate Professor of Practice / Clinical Pharmacy Specialist
North Dakota State, Department of Pharmacy Practice, University College of Health Professions

Michelle B. McElhannon, PharmD

IPPE Experiences, Clinical Pharmacist – DSMES
Public Service Assistant, Division of Experience Programs, University of Georgia College of Pharmacy

M. Shawn McFarland, PharmD, FCCP, BCACP

National Clinical Pharmacy Practice Program Manager
Clinical Pharmacy Practice Office Pharmacy Benefits Management Services
Veterans Health Administration, Washington, DC

Jeffery L. Olson, PharmD, MBA, BCPS, BCACP

Pharmacy Operations Director
Intermountain Healthcare

DOI 10.37573/9781585286928.FM

Ashley Marie Parrott, PharmD, MBA, BCPS, BCACP

Manager, Ambulatory Clinical Pharmacy Services
Parkview Health, Department of Pharmacy

Jennifer Reiter, PharmD, MBA, BCACP

Pharmacy Manager–Ambulatory Care
Indiana University Health Southern Indiana Physicians

Eve M. Segal, PharmD, BCOP

Lead Clinical Pharmacist, Hematology/Oncology
University of Washington Medical Center/Seattle Cancer Care Alliance

Jessica W. Skelley, PharmD, BCACP

Associate Professor of Pharmacy Practice Adjunct Faculty, St. Vincent's East Family Medicine Residency Program
Department of Pharmacy Practice
Samford University

Andrew S. Tenpas, PharmD

Clinical Assistant Professor
Department of Pharmacy Practice, Texas A&M Irma Lerma Rangel College of Pharmacy

Laura Traynor, PharmD, BCACP, AE-C

Ambulatory (MTM) Pharmacist – Diabetes and Endocrinology Clinic
Hennepin Healthcare, Minneapolis, MN

Angelina Vascimini, PharmD

Assistant Professor
Department of Pharmacotherapeutics and Clinical Research
University of South Florida Taneja College of Pharmacy

Felix K. Yam, PharmD, M.A.S., BCPS, BCCP

Associate Clinical Professor
Division of Clinical Pharmacy, UC San Diego Skaggs School of Pharmacy and Pharmaceutical Sciences

REVIEWERS

Jillanne Schulte Wall, J.D.

Senior Director, Health and Regulatory Policy
Office of Government Relations
ASHP

Jennifer Reiter, PharmD, MBA, BCACP

Pharmacy Manager–Ambulatory Care
Indiana University Health Southern Indiana Physicians

Ashley Marie Parrott, PharmD, MBA, BCPS, BCACP*

Manager, Ambulatory Clinical Pharmacy Services
Parkview Health, Department of Pharmacy

*Dr. Parrott also authored the clinical vignettes.

DOI 10.37573/9781585286928.FM

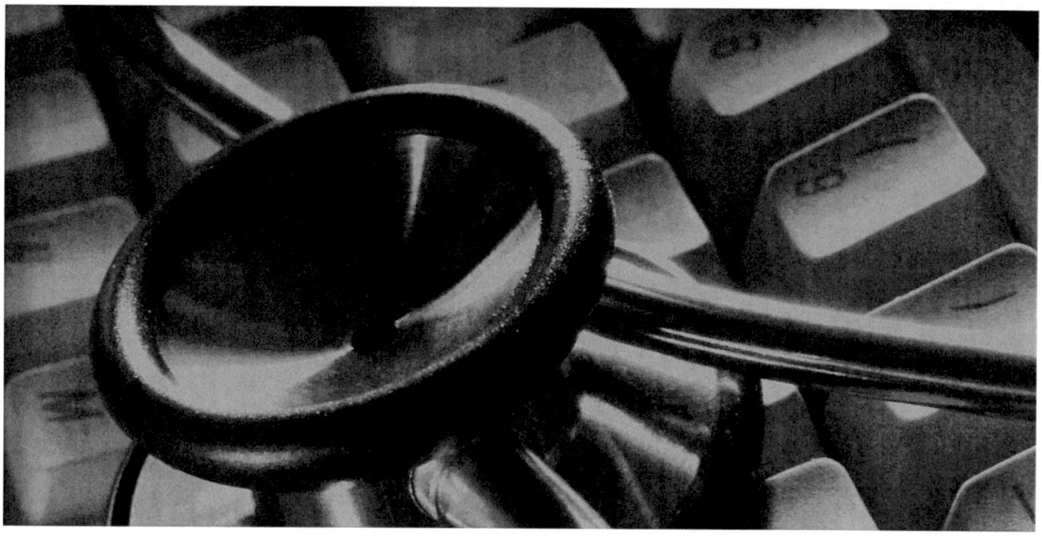

SECTION 1
Foundational Information for Understanding Telehealth Pharmacy Practice

Jessica W. Skelley, Ashley Marie Parrott, Joe Lassiter, and Laura Traynor

CHAPTER 1
Exploring the History and Literature of Telehealth

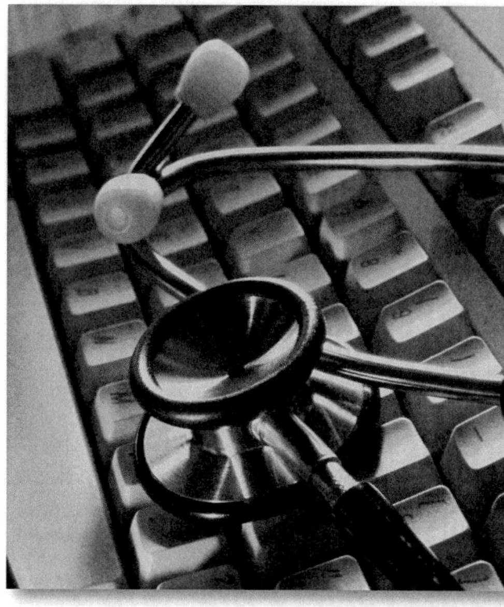

HISTORY IN MEDICAL PRACTICE—TELEHEALTH THEN AND NOW

Telehealth has been defined as the use of telecommunication technologies to deliver distanced healthcare.[1] Stated another way, telehealth is remote care delivered via technology. While often used interchangeably with the term *telemedicine*, telehealth is typically utilized when describing direct clinical services. Telehealth is a broader term encompassing a wide array of health-related services delivered at a distance, including patient care, patient and provider education, and remote monitoring.[2] Telemedicine and other ancillary telemedicine services have been in existence for a century, with the first case documented in the 1920s when medical specialists on land were connected via radio to those with medical emergencies at sea.[3] Since then, telehealth has undergone several periods of growth and evolution. Telehealth pharmacy practice is simply focused on titling for pharmacists engaged in this remote platform for patient care activities.

Within the last several decades, early applications of telehealth worked to expand access to care in prisons, military locations, and rural areas.[4] Hospitals also began to adopt telehealth, with one of the first documented uses being in the 1950s–1960s when the Nebraska Psychiatric Institute and Norfolk State Hospital established a closed-circuit television link to facilitate psychiatric consultations.[5] Additionally, practice areas such as dermatology and psychiatry have been early adopters of telemedicine, showing positive outcomes such as high rates of agreement between diagnoses made both in person and during telehealth visits and high satisfaction rates.[5]

While telehealth was initially considered primarily as a potential tool to improve patient access to care, focus is now shifting to the potential for telehealth to reduce costs.[6,7] Healthcare organizations have recognized that by facilitating access to timely services, overall healthcare expenditures may be reduced if patient utilization of hospital admissions, emergency room services, and other high-cost services are lowered. While telehealth was initially used primarily to address more acute issues such as stroke, a notable shift has taken place toward leveraging telehealth services to manage chronic disease states.[8] As technology is increasingly available to assist providers in monitoring and caring for patients, it is likely that the role of telehealth in caring for chronic conditions, that historically necessitated an office visit for purposes such as lab collection and vital sign information, will expand.

DOI 10.37573/9781585286928.001

Telehealth Challenges Throughout Time

In order for telehealth to achieve its full potential, it must not only be incorporated into hospital and outpatient practices, but also address the six domains of quality of care defined by the Institution of Medicine: safe, effective, patient-centered, timely, efficient, and equitable.[2] Significant challenges stand in the way of achieving this goal, although much progress has been made in many areas over the last decade.

In some states, complications surrounding state licensure and practice laws can create roadblocks for the effective utilization of telehealth.[9] Patients may not be able to receive remote care from a provider that is not currently licensed in the state where the patient is located. Additionally, some states have practice laws that prevent providers from prescribing medications in conjunction with a telehealth visit, limiting the care that the patient can receive.[1,9] Credentialing issues can also be difficult, with practices that have multiple locations and multiple providers engaging in telehealth. Moreover, questions over liability related to telehealth continue in the medical community at large.

Reimbursement has been frequently named as one of the most significant challenges to telehealth expansion and sustainability.[10,11] In a study from 2017 that surveyed 104 healthcare organizations, over half of respondents indicated that reimbursement limitations minimized their ability to further expand access to telehealth services for patients.[1] Private insurances offer varying levels of reimbursement, similar to Medicaid. Medicare has historically been the most limiting in terms of reimbursement for telehealth services, although recent improvements have been seen beginning in 2020 in the wake of COVID-19 and the need to rapidly expand telehealth services to the vulnerable Medicare population.

Access to technology necessary to engage in pharmacy telehealth services is also a challenge for some patients. While a 2021 report stated that approximately 93% of American adults currently have access to the Internet, only 75% of the 65 and older population use the Internet—representing the lowest percentage of any age group.[12] In rural areas access to high-speed Internet can be difficult, which may impact patients' abilities to engage in video telehealth visits. A 2018 report found that 58% of Americans living in rural areas found access to high-speed Internet problematic.[13] Lastly, socioeconomic factors may impact telehealth uptake due to access issues, with underserved patients using video telehealth services less than other groups.[11]

Some reports have cited provider unwillingness to adopt telehealth as a primary driver for its historically limited uptake.[10] This hesitancy may be due to lack of training and familiarity with telehealth, as well as to the perception that it may be ineffective or unsafe or that it will negatively impact practice workflow and efficiency.[10] Clinicians often receive only limited exposure to telehealth in their formal education, necessitating further professional development once they are out in practice.[10,14,15] Lastly, providers' concerns regarding surrounding clinical challenges such as the ability to perform a quality physical examination should be considered.[9] Provider uptake of telehealth pharmacy practice models may be impacted by the presence of a "provider champion" to advocate for its use and by the provision of incentives to participate in education and development activities related to telehealth.[11,16]

Patient uptake can also be a challenge in the expansion of telehealth. Like providers, patients have expressed a concern about the provider's potential lack of ability to perform a sufficient physical exam, as well as about the privacy of the visit, depending on their physical location.[17] Older patients experience barriers such as lack of desire to participate in telehealth services, technical literacy challenges, and perception of increased cost of care in the event their insurance does not cover these services.[10] The patient–provider relationship may also be harder to establish in a telehealth environment, as these visits often can occur with providers the patient has not had a previously established relationship with, which may increase care fragmentation.[10]

Finally, healthcare technology and electronic health records (EHRs) pose various challenges, which will be further explored in Chapter 3 of the present section.

RECENT DEVELOPMENTS IN TELEHEALTH

Expansion of Telehealth Services

Many large healthcare organizations have seen a significant growth in their utilization of pharmacy telehealth services over the past decade. Starting in 2016, Kaiser Permanente reported that their virtual services exceeded their provision of in-person visits.[18] While they noted a higher overall volume of patient visits in those organizations utilizing telehealth when compared with those using in-person visits, this statistic did not necessarily correspond to higher healthcare expenditures.[19] The Department of Veterans Affairs health system has also escalated their use of telehealth services, reporting a 2,000-fold increase in telehealth over a 20-year period.[20]

COVID-19 Related Changes

In 2017, the Department of Health and Human Services estimated that over half of all healthcare institutions in the United States used some form of telehealth.[21] This number is likely significantly higher in the wake of COVID-19, as in 2020 many institutions and organizations were forced to engage in rapid uptake of these services to deliver care to a population under stay-at-home orders. One organization reported that following the initial COVID-19 outbreak, the portion of telehealth visits jumped within a 4-week period from <1% of total visits to approximately 70% of total visits.[22] Other healthcare organizations described rapid scale-up of telehealth services to various patient populations, including adolescents, obstetrics, mental health, and geriatric patients.[14,23-26]

COVID-19 is not the first crisis to precipitate an increase in telehealth offerings. Notably, Hurricanes Harvey and Irma in 2017, the 2003 SARS pandemic in China, and severe droughts and bush fires in Australia in 2019–2020 all also resulted in increased telehealth provisions.[10] Regardless, outside of these emergency situations, overall uptake to telehealth within the larger healthcare community has been slow. Relying on sporadic uptake of telehealth in times of a pandemic or other global crisis will not result in long-term changes to the healthcare landscape. In order to provide for long-term sustainability of telehealth services following the expansion related to COVID-19, consideration should be given to needs related to providing education, developing reimbursement models, improving technology, integrating telehealth workflow into daily provision of care to patients, and empowering patients.[10,14,15,22,25]

Integration of Wearable Medical Devices with Telehealth

Technology advances, including remote patient monitoring (RPM), video and audio technologies, and mobile health, have resulted in new and innovative ways to engage in patient care.[1] Remote patient monitoring involves patient health data being reported, collected, transmitted, and evaluated through electronic devices such as mobile devices, smartphone apps, and wearable technology. These devices can collect and transfer data such as vital signs, send patients reminders to weigh themselves or take medications, and track data such as blood glucose.[1,27,28] While data have provided mixed results of their clinical outcomes and long-term efficacy, patients report overall increased engagement and may see improved outcomes with reduced costs of care.[1,27-29,30-33]

ESTABLISHED POSITIVE TELEHEALTH PRACTICE OUTCOMES

Even prior to the onset of the COVID-19 pandemic, many organizations had been working on implementing a telehealth strategy that would align with their goals and priorities. The pandemic has drastically accelerated the need for both telehealth options and legislation to support telehealth services and reimbursement. Telehealth pharmacy practice models may vary based on location, available resources, patient population, and service provided. In the following pages, we explore literature related to potential benefits seen with telehealth services (often compared to standard or usual care) in both a general context and the pharmacy-specific literature.

General Literature Establishing Positive Outcomes

A 2018 rapid review published by Shigekawa and associates assessed systematic reviews and meta-analyses that were published from January 2004 to May 2018 related to telehealth services that allowed direct interaction between patients and providers. This article reviewed studies that included either adults or children involved in telehealth care for either a disease or condition, including diagnosis and/or treatment. The accepted modalities for telehealth care included live video-conferencing, asynchronous store-and-forward platforms, telephone (excluding disease management delivered by nurses), email, chat, or text. The intervention group was compared to usual care (in-person treatment). Outcomes were variable but often included clinical outcomes, process outcomes, and/or healthcare utilization. Studies included in the rapid review addressed diagnosis and/or treatment in telemental health, telerehabilitation, teledermatology, teleconsultation, oral anticoagulation management, nutrition, and diabetic foot ulcer treatment. Based on their evaluation of the included studies, the authors concluded that, for the conditions or disease states evaluated, telehealth was equivalent to in-person care in most cases. The authors were not able to draw conclusions on whether the use of telehealth services impacted the use of other services—whether an increase or a decrease in utilization.[34]

A systematic review by DeNicola and colleagues addressed a different specialty than that seen in the rapid review by Shigekawa and associates. DeNicola and colleagues sought to review the effectiveness of telehealth to improve outcomes in obstetrics and gynecology. These authors defined telehealth as including the use of technology to enhance healthcare, such as virtual visits, remote patient monitoring, and mobile apps or text messaging that could use either synchronous or asynchronous communication. The authors sought to address four areas within the framework of this systematic review. The questions all related to assessing if telehealth served as either an effective adjunct or an alternative to standard of care for improving outcomes related to four different areas: family planning, low-risk obstetrics, high-risk obstetrics, and gynecologic outcomes. Studies that included men or children were excluded. Those studies that only evaluated telehealth outcomes related to access and/or patient or provider accessibility and satisfaction were also excluded, as were studies that included telephone-only or website-only interventions and studies that focused on fertility and fertility tracking. Ultimately, 47 studies were included in the final evaluation, which had 31,967 participants. Overall, the authors concluded that telehealth interventions were associated with improved obstetric outcomes in several areas, including perinatal smoking cessation, breastfeeding, early access to medical abortion services, and scheduled optimization for high-risk obstetrics. The review suggested that specific interventions (text messaging and remote monitoring) may have had more benefit. The authors suggested additional studies to further examine the impact of specific technologies that had been integrated into telehealth care for patients of obstetrics and gynecology.[35]

Wu and colleagues completed a systematic review and meta-analysis to evaluate clinical outcomes of telehealth compared to usual care for managing diabetes. The authors included randomized controlled trials (RCTs) that reported the clinical outcomes of adult patients with either type 1 or type 2 diabetes. Telehealth intervention was defined as including at least one of the following: tele-education, telemonitoring, teleconsultation, and telecase management. To be included, trials needed to have greater than 100 participants and at least six months of follow-up. Trials involving gestational diabetes were not included. A total of 19 RCTs were included in the final analysis, with 6294 participants (3269 of whom received a telehealth intervention, while 3025 received usual care). The authors concluded that there is an association between use of telehealth and improved clinical outcomes for patients with diabetes. Overall, with telehealth, both blood pressure and glycemic control showed improvement, while no difference was found in change in body mass index. Patients with a hemoglobin A1c of at least 9% may see more benefit. In addition, touchpoints of at least six times per year may result in greater benefit.[36]

Pharmacy-Specific Literature Evaluating Positive Outcomes

An early telehealth study published in 2003 by Chan and colleagues demonstrated the use of an Internet-based store-and-forward video home telehealth system in pediatric patients with asthma compared to standard in-office care and education. In this study, 10 children participated in the virtual education group and were asked twice per week to submit their electronic asthma symptom diary, along with a video of peak flow meter use and controller medication use. Twice every week a pharmacist would review the videos and the asthma symptom diary and provide patients with feedback. Patients also had access to an educational website. Outcomes assessed included patient adherence, various markers of disease control, parent satisfaction, and asthma knowledge retention. While there were no differences in outcome measures between the virtual and in-office group for the total study period, this study did demonstrate the feasibility of using virtual education and assessment methods in pediatric patients with asthma.[37]

A 2015 study by Singh and associates evaluated the use of clinical video telehealth (CVT) technology to optimize the clinical pharmacy specialist (CPS) staffing model within the Virginia Maryland healthcare system (VAMHCS) for anticoagulation visits. The patient care CVT system had one telehealth station at the patient site and another at the provider site. Patients were scheduled for 20-minute appointments. At the patient site, nursing staff assessed vital signs and performed a point-of-care (POC) International Normalized Ratio (INR) testing. Then, a telehealth technician ensured that the patient was appropriately set up with the CVT equipment and was available to assist in physical assessments if needed. The technician also scheduled follow-up appointments. The CPS was located at the provider site and performed the clinical components of the visit, including gathering patient history, evaluating the patient's warfarin regimen, and developing an appropriate pharmacotherapeutic plan for the patient's anticoagulation. Outcomes included the use of CVT on patients' INR values (time in therapeutic range [TTR]) and patient satisfaction following six months of the service. TTR was found to be comparable before and after CVT implementation (mean ± *SD* of 76.4% ± 18.8% vs 80.8% ± 16.1%). Patient satisfaction was found to be a mean ± *SD* of 4.77 ± 0.14 (maximum of 5), with a survey response rate of over 80%. The authors concluded that the use of CVT maintained high-quality anticoagulation services and patient satisfaction while optimizing the staffing of the CPS.[38]

Shane-McWhorter et al. assessed clinical outcomes along with disease state knowledge, adherence, and self-efficacy for patients with diabetes using telemonitoring devices. A total of 150 patients were included in the analysis, with 75 patients in the pharmacist-led telemonitoring group and 75 patients receiving usual care across four federally qualified community health centers in Utah. Patients were included in the study if they were adult patients with type 2 diabetes (with or without hypertension) and a hemoglobin A1c value greater than 7%. Patients needed to be willing to participate and follow instructions as well as use the telemonitoring equipment. Patients did need either telephone or Internet access to be included in the study. Patients in the telemonitoring group used either a remote monitoring device or an interactive voice response (IVR) system. Both pieces of technology were from the same vendor and allowed patients to be monitored in an asynchronous manner. Data were immediately accessible via a secure website. Telemonitoring took place Monday through Friday and typically lasted 5 to 10 minutes. The pharmacist would review data in the secure portal several times each day and reach out to patients with out-of-range blood glucose values or blood pressure values. The intervention group had a decrease in HbA1c of 2.07% ($p<0.001$) from baseline to the end of study, which was significantly greater compared to the 0.66% reduction ($p=0.006$) in the usual care group. The HbA1c reduction did not differ significantly by modality used (remote monitoring device vs IVR) in the intervention group. Blood pressure, low-density lipoprotein (LDL) cholesterol, and body mass index (BMI) did not differ significantly between the two groups. Self-efficacy, diabetes, and hypertension knowledge all improved in the intervention group compared to baseline ($p \le 0.01$ for all). There was improvement in adherence to hypertension medications in the intervention group compared to baseline (p <0.001), but there was not statistically significant improvement in adherence to diabetes medications. The authors concluded that pharmacy telehealth services for monitoring clinical parameters, medication management, and disease-specific education have the potential to improve clinical outcomes.[39]

In 2021, Seamon and colleagues published a study on a telemedicine initiative focusing on a rural population with uncontrolled diabetes. A total of 64 patients were included in the program, with 46 patients remaining in the telemedicine program for a sufficient period of time to obtain a postcontact HbA1c. For those 46 patients, there was a significant reduction in mean HbA1c of 1.15 ($t = -3.5$, p <0.01) compared with baseline HbA1c values. The most common intervention categories included addressing medication access concerns, titrating insulin therapy, providing education, and making appointments or addressing labs that were due. The authors concluded that a pharmacist-led telemedicine program for rural patients with uncontrolled diabetes was associated with a reduction in HbA1c.[40]

Niznik and associates conducted a systematic review and meta-analysis to determine the impact of clinical pharmacist-led telemedicine interventions on various outcomes, including disease management, patient self-management, and adherence. Studies were included if they involved a pharmacist as part of the care delivery (whether the sole provider or part of a team) and used telemedicine technology as defined by the American Telemedicine Association. A focus was given to articles on the outpatient and ambulatory care setting and those articles that used a comparator group for measurable, clinical outcomes. Articles focusing on dispensing or preparing medications were excluded. Thirty-four articles met the inclusion criteria in the analysis. The authors noted that studies reporting clinical outcomes for chronic disease management studies had an overall positive rate of 67.8% (19 of 28). Studies assessing patient self-management outcomes had an overall positive rate of 100% but included a small number of studies ($n = 2$). Studies evaluating adherence outcomes had an overall positive rate of 62.5% (five of eight). It was not possible to compile results into a meta-analysis due to the heterogeneity of study designs and outcomes. The authors noted two overall themes: that most telemedicine interventions resulted in a positive impact on outcomes and that scheduled models of care (i.e., scheduled appointments) were utilized most often.[41]

The preceding content explored various aspects of telehealth that were both nonpharmacy specific and pharmacy specific. Literature reviews were outlined that establish the use of telehealth as a reasonable adjunct or an alternative to standard of care in various specialty areas to provide similar or improved patient outcomes. Additional literature outlined various examples of telehealth pharmacy practice initiatives and the success of those models. For more information, review Section 4: Tracking Metrics for Improved Care Quality, Increased Care Access, and Patient Experience, which contains more examples from the literature demonstrating the effectiveness of telehealth services as well as additional aspects such as patient experience and improving access to care.

CONCLUSION

Telehealth offers the opportunity to expand the reach of medicine while providing a potential for reduced costs alongside increased quality. While challenges remain concerning reimbursement, patient access, and other factors, great improvements have been made in the scale and provision of telehealth services over the past decade, and especially in the past year owing to the COVID-19 pandemic. In order to sustain this rapid growth, consideration must be given to the long-term sustainability of these clinical services and to support the clinicians who will engage in telehealth pharmacy practice with appropriate training, education, and backup as they continually transform their practice to meet the needs of a changing population. Further studies assessing various models and modalities for delivery of pharmacist-led telehealth services are needed.

REFERENCES

1. Catalyst NEJM. What Is Telehealth? *NEJM Catalyst*. **https://catalyst.nejm.org/doi/full/10.1056/CAT.18.0268**. Published February 1, 2018. Accessed May 16, 2021. **https://catalyst.nejm.org/doi/full/10.1056/CAT.18.0268**.
2. Schwamm LH. Telehealth: Seven strategies to successfully implement disruptive technology and transform health care. *Health Affairs*. 2014;33(2):200-206. doi:10.1377/hlthaff.2013.1021.
3. Winters SR. Diagnosis by wireless. *Sci Am*. 1921;124(24):465.
4. Bashshur RL, Reardon TG, Shannon GW. Telemedicine: A new health care delivery system. *Annual Reviews in Public Health* 2000;21(1):613-637. doi: 10.1146/annurev.publhealth.21.1.613.
5. Board on Health Care Services; Institute of Medicine. The role of telehealth in an evolving health care environment: Workshop summary. Washington, DC: National Academies Press (US); 2012 November 20:3; The evolution of telehealth: Where have we been and where are we going? **https://www.ncbi.nlm.nih.gov/books/NBK207141**. Accessed May 16, 2021.
6. United States Senate Committee on Finance. Bipartisan chronic care working group policy options document. December 2015. **https://www.finance.senate.gov/imo/media/doc/CCWG%20Policy%20Options%20Paper1.pdf**. Accessed May 16, 2021.
7. Mistry H. Systematic review of studies of the cost-effectiveness of telemedicine and telecare. Changes in the economic evidence over twenty years. *J Telemed Telecare*. 2012;18(1):1-6. doi: 10.1258/jtt.2011.110505.
8. Levine SR, Gorman M. "Telestroke": The application of telemedicine for stroke. *Stroke* 1999;30: 464-469. **https://doi.org/10.1161/01.STR.30.2.464**.
9. Dorsey ER, Topol EJ. State of telehealth. *N Engl J Med*. 2016;375(2):154-161. doi:10.1056/nejmra1601705.
10. Smith AC, Thomas E, Snoswell CL, et al. Telehealth for global emergencies: Implications for coronavirus disease 2019 (COVID-19). *J Telemed Telecare*. 2020;26(5):309-313. doi:10.1177/1357633x20916567.
11. Kvedar J, Coye MJ, Everett W. Connected health: A review of technologies and strategies to improve patient care with telemedicine and telehealth. *Health Affairs*. 2014;33(2):194-199. doi:10.1377/hlthaff.2013.0992.
12. Demographics of Internet and Home Broadband Usage in the United States. Pew Research Center: Internet, Science & Tech. **https://www.pewresearch.org/internet/fact-sheet/internet-broadband**. Published April 8, 2021. Accessed May 16, 2021.
13. Anderson M. For 24% of rural Americans, high-speed internet is a major problem. Pew Research Center. **https://www.pewresearch.org/fact-tank/2018/09/10/about-a-quarter-of-rural-americans-say-access-to-high-speed-internet-is-a-major-problem**. Published August 21, 2020. Accessed May 16, 2021.
14. Thomas EE, Haydon HM, Mehrotra A, et al. Building on the momentum: Sustaining telehealth beyond COVID-19. *J Telemed Telecare*. 2020. doi:10.1177/1357633x20960638.
15. Wijesooriya NR, Mishra V, Brand PLP, Rubin BK. COVID-19 and telehealth, education, and research adaptations. *Paediatr Respir Rev*. 2020;(35):38-42. **https://doi.org/10.1016/j.prrv.2020.06.009**.
16. Ellimoottil C, An L, Moyer M, et al. Challenges and opportunities faced by large health systems implementing telehealth. *Health Affairs*. 2018;37(12):1955-1959. doi:10.1377/hlthaff.2018.05099.
17. Powell RE, Henstenburg JM, Cooper G, et al. Patient perceptions of telehealth primary care video visits. *Ann Fam Med*. 2017;15(3):225-229. doi: **https://doi.org/10.1370/afm.2095**.
18. Advisory Board. A milestone: Kaiser now interacts more with patients virtually than in-person. Daily Briefing. October 13, 2016. **https://www.advisory.com/daily-briefing/2016/10/13/kaiser-telehealth**. Accessed May 16, 2021.
19. Pearl R. Kaiser Permanente Northern California: Current experiences with internet, mobile, and video technologies. *Health Aff (Millwood)*. 2014;33:251-257. doi: 10.1377/hlthaff.2013.1005.
20. Darkins A. The growth of telehealth services in the Veterans Health Administration between 1994 and 2014: A study in the diffusion of Innovation. *Telemed e-Health*. 2014;20(9):761-768. doi:10.1089/tmj.2014.0143.
21. Tuckson RV, Edmunds M, Hodgkins ML. Telehealth. *N Engl J Med*. 2017;377(16):1585-1592. doi:10.1056/nejmsr1503323.

22. Wosik J, Fudim M, Cameron B, et al. Telehealth transformation: COVID-19 and the rise of virtual care. *J Am Med Inform Assoc.* 2020;27(6):957-962. **https://doi.org/10.1093/jamia/ocaa067**.

23. Wood SM, White K, Peebles R, et al. Outcomes of a rapid adolescent telehealth scale-up during the COVID-19 Pandemic. *J Adolesc Health* 2020;67(2):172-178. **https://doi.org/10.1016/j.jadohealth.2020.05.025**.

24. Zhou X, Snoswell CL, Harding LE, et al. The role of telehealth in reducing the mental health burden from COVID-19. *Telemedicine and e-Health.* 2020;26(4):377-379. doi:10.1089/tmj.2020.0068.

25. Monaghesh E, Hajizadeh A. The role of telehealth during COVID-19 outbreak: A systematic review based on current evidence. *BMC Public Health.* 2020;20(1). doi:10.1186/s12889-020-09301-4.

26. Fryer K, Delgado A, Foti T, et al. Implementation of obstetric telehealth during COVID-19 and beyond. *Matern Child Health Jl.* 2020;24(9):1104-1110. doi:10.1007/s10995-020-02967-7.

27. Greenwood DA, Young HM, Quinn CC. Telehealth remote monitoring systematic review. *J Diabetes Sci Tech.* 2014;8(2):378-389. doi:10.1177/1932296813519311.

28. Lee PA, Greenfield G, Pappas Y. The impact of telehealth remote patient monitoring on glycemic control in type 2 diabetes: A systematic review and meta-analysis of systematic reviews of randomised controlled trials. *BMC Health Serv Res.* 2018;18(1). doi:10.1186/s12913-018-3274-8. **https://bmchealthservres.biomedcentral.com/articles/10.1186/s12913-018-3274-8**.

29. Vegesna A, Tran M, Angelaccio M, Arcona S. Remote patient monitoring via non-invasive digital technologies: A systematic review. *Telemed J e-Health.* 2017;23(1):3-17. doi:10.1089/tmj.2016.0051.

30. Kamei T, Kanamori T, Yamamoto Y, Edirippulige S. The use of wearable devices in chronic disease management to enhance adherence and improve telehealth outcomes: A systematic review and meta-analysis. *J Telemed Telecare.* 2020. doi:10.1177/1357633x20937573.

31. Ding X, Clifton D, Ji N, et al. Wearable sensing and telehealth technology with potential applications in the coronavirus pandemic. *IEEE Rev Biomed Eng.* 2021;14:48-70. doi: 10.1109/RBME.2020.2992838.

32. Wang C, Lu W, Narayanan MR, et al. Low-power technologies for wearable telecare and telehealth systems: A review. *Biomed Eng Letters* 2015;5:1-9.

33. Dang S, Dimmick S, Kelkar G. Evaluating the evidence base for the use of home telehealth remote monitoring in elderly with heart failure. *Telemed e-Health.* 2009;15(8):783-796. doi:10.1089/tmj.2009.0028.

34. Shigekawa E, Fix M, Corbett G, et al. The current state of telehealth evidence: A rapid review. *Health Aff (Millwood).* 2018;37(12):1975-1982. doi: 10.1377/hlthaff.2018.05132.

35. DeNicola N, Grossman D, Marko K, et al. Telehealth interventions to improve obstetric and gynecologic health outcomes. *Obstet Gynecol.* 2020 Feb;135(2):371-382. doi: 10.1097/AOG.0000000000003646.

36. Wu CW, Wu Z, Yang L, et al. Evaluation of the clinical outcomes of telehealth for managing diabetes: A PRISMA-compliant meta-analysis. *Medicine (Baltimore).* 2018 Oct;97(43):e12962. doi: 10.1097/MD.0000000000012962.

37. Chan DS, Callahan CW, Sheets SJ, et al. An internet-based store-and-forward video home telehealth system for improving asthma outcomes in children. *Am J Health Syst Pharm.* 2003; 1;60(19):1976-1981. doi: 10.1093/ajhp/60.19.1976.

38. Singh LG, Accursi M, Black KK. Implementation and outcomes of a pharmacist-managed clinical video telehealth anticoagulation clinic. *Am J Health Syst Pharm.* 2015 Jan 1;72(1):70-73. doi: 10.2146/ajhp130750.

39. Shane-McWhorter L, McAdam-Marx C, Lenert L, et al. Pharmacist-provided diabetes management and education via a telemonitoring program. *J Am Pharm Assoc.* 2003;Sep-Oct 2015;55(5):516-526. doi: 10.1331/JAPhA.2015.14285.

40. Seamon G, Caron O, Jiang A, et al. Pharmacist-led phone call initiative targeting hemoglobin A1c levels in patients with uncontrolled diabetes. *J Am Coll Clin Pharm.* 2021;1-7.

41. Niznik JD, He H, Kane-Gill SL. Impact of clinical pharmacist services delivered via telemedicine in the outpatient or ambulatory care setting: A systematic review. *Res Social Adm Pharm.* 2018 Aug;14(8):707-717. doi: 10.1016/j.sapharm.2017.10.011.

CHAPTER 2 Establishing the Definitions for Telehealth

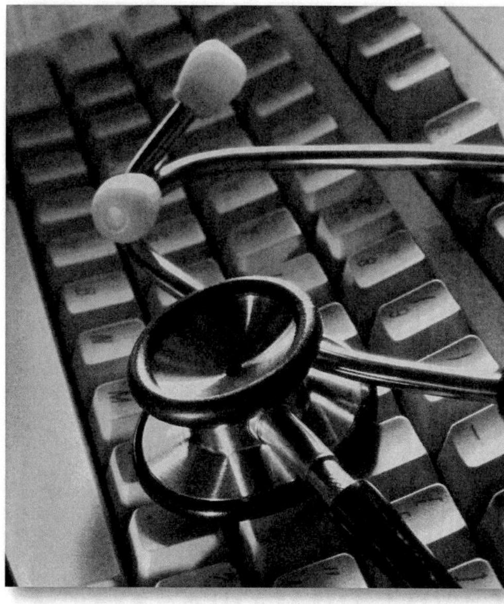

Before we approach the discussion about the integration of telehealth into contemporary pharmacy practice, it is important that we discuss the terminology to understand the background and application of the various terms associated with this treatment modality. The terminology discussed in this chapter will apply to subsequent sections and chapters of this text and will be used as a framework to understand how these technologies apply to pharmacy practice. In defining the terminology, resources from several sources were considered, including payers (e.g., U.S. Centers for Medicare & Medicaid Services [CMS]);[1] practitioner organizations (e.g., American Medical Association [AMA]);[2] educational organizations (e.g., American Board of Telehealth);[3] trade organizations (e.g., American Telemedicine Association [ATA]);[4] coalitions (e.g., National Consortium of Telehealth Resource Centers [NCTRC]);[5] and governmental bodies (e.g., The Office of the National Coordinator for Health Information Technology [ONC]).[6-8] Although all resources reviewed had their own perspectives, based on the mission and purpose of the organization itself, common elements of the definitions were synthesized to develop and expand the definitions and terminology in this chapter.

As a developing modality for delivering treatment—which was propelled into increased deployment and use by the Coronavirus disease 2019 (COVID-19) pandemic—the definitions for telehealth and associated terms are somewhat dynamic and have the potential to adjust over time. As telehealth shifts from a modality deployed to address a public health crisis to a treatment delivery option widely available for patient care, education, and care coordination, the terminology will perhaps adjust to new phrases, definitions, or standardization across platforms.

TELEHEALTH

A succinct and practical definition of telehealth is the use of telecommunication technologies to deliver distanced healthcare. Another way of stating the definition is that telehealth is remote care delivered via technology. Now let's separate that definition into its components and discuss what is meant by healthcare, the concept of distanced care, and, finally, what technologies are utilized.

First, the term *healthcare* is used broadly to describe any aspect of patient care, whether it be administrative, population-based, or direct. Most commonly, telehealth is used in reference to direct patient care from a provider to patient and/or their caregiver(s). However, during the pandemic, telehealth has increasingly been utilized as a modality for delivery of public health initiatives, such as education of populations and coordination of immunization campaigns.

Second, a key aspect of telehealth is that it is delivered remotely, over a distance. That

DOI 10.37573/9781585286928.002

distance may vary with need. For example, a pharmacist located at an academic medical center may be counseling a patient who lives close by, such as in a suburban area of the same city. Another example, frequently cited for telehealth prior to the pandemic, is to extend care to rural and underserved areas in which the patient could be hundreds of miles away from the practitioner delivering the care. The essential element is that the practitioner and the patient, or audience, are in dissimilar locations, thus necessitating remote care.

Lastly, healthcare providers utilize various telecommunications technologies to deliver remote or distanced care. Telecommunications refers to the electronic exchange of information over a distance. From a technical standpoint, a telecommunications arrangement is made up of two or more stations with transmitter and receiver devices.[9,10] Modern telecommunications devices include telephones, radio, fiber optics, satellites, and the Internet. For the purposes of this textbook, we will focus on telehealth being delivered via telephone and via the Internet because those are the two most common modalities in contemporary practice.[11] Additionally, the term *telehealth pharmacy practice* (or *service*) will be used to separate focused remote activities from the other similar terminology to be discussed in this chapter and allow for breadth of practice variations from pharmacists provided remotely.

TELEMEDICINE

If telehealth is defined as the use of telecommunication technologies to deliver distanced healthcare, what then is telemedicine? In discussions with colleagues at your practice sites, and even in podium presentations at national conferences, these terms may be used interchangeably. However, for the purpose of our discussion in this text, we define telemedicine as a service provided separately from telehealth. Similar to telehealth, telemedicine aims to address a patient's health status via interactive communication between the patient and the provider at a distant site.[12] Therefore, telemedicine can be considered a subset of telehealth focusing on the delivery of medicine using telecommunication technology. In contrast to telemedicine, telehealth is a broader term encompassing not only the practice of medicine, but also public health initiatives, such as education and training. In considering the definition of telemedicine in contrast to telehealth, we can also consider the practitioners utilizing these tools. By definition, telehealth can be utilized by any healthcare practitioner, including public health professionals. In contrast, telemedicine should be considered the domain of medicine practitioners licensed to practice medicine, such as physicians, nurse practitioners, and physician assistants. Telemedicine is viewed by payers as a cost-effective alternative to the standard method of providing medical care (i.e., in-person consultations between provider and patient).[12]

REMOTE PATIENT MONITORING

Remote patient monitoring (RPM) refers to the collection and transmission of patient data from outside the health system (i.e., outside of an acute or ambulatory patient care setting); these data are typically collected in an asynchronous manner. Devices or applications that collect patient clinical data (e.g., weight, blood pressure, pulse oximetry, respiratory rate) or measure therapy response are utilized at the remote location. The information collected and transmitted in RPM can subsequently be used in clinical decision making and care follow-up.[13] For regulatory and reimbursement purposes, remote patient monitoring is not considered telemedicine per se; however, the follow-up care delivered as a result of the clinical data collected via RPM may be conducted via telemedicine technology. For example, a home health patient on intravenous antibiotic therapy is being monitored at home utilizing devices that capture temperature, blood pressure, and pulse oximetry. The triage nurse at the health system's infectious disease clinic notes a worsening of the patient systems upon review of their clinical data from the remote monitoring devices. Due to the concerning clinical information, the triage nurse schedules a video visit between the resident infectious diseases physician and the patient, together with their caregiver. The first part of this scenario is RPM: asynchronous data are collected and transmitted to the remote care team. When the video visit takes place between physician and patient, and caregiver, this is considered telemedicine.

TELEPHARMACY

As is true of the terms *telehealth* and *telemedicine*, the terms *telehealth* and *telepharmacy* are frequently used interchangeably among colleagues in a pharmacy practice setting. However, for the purposes of this text, we consider telepharmacy a distinct term and a distinct delivery of pharmacy services. What is telepharmacy? The August 2020 Model State Pharmacy Act and Model Rules of the National Association of Boards of Pharmacy (NABP) define telepharmacy as "the practice of pharmacy by registered pharmacies and pharmacists located within US jurisdictions through the use of telepharmacy technologies between a licensee and patients or their agents at distances that are located within US jurisdictions. The practice of telepharmacy is deemed to occur within the jurisdiction in which the patient is located and the jurisdiction(s) in which the pharmacist and, if applicable, pharmacy are located; therefore, such practice will be subject to the pharmacy practice regulations of all jurisdictions' Boards of Pharmacy."[14] The American Society of Health-System Pharmacy (ASHP) defines telepharmacy as "a method used in pharmacy practice in which a pharmacist utilizes telecommunications technology to oversee aspects of pharmacy operations or provide patient-care services." Further, ASHP states that "telepharmacy operations and services may include, but are not limited to, drug review and monitoring, dispensing, sterile and nonsterile compounding verification, medication therapy management (MTM), patient assessment, patient counseling, clinical consultation, outcomes assessment, decision support, and drug information."[15] As we can see from these definitions, telepharmacy can be considered a subset of telehealth for the provision of pharmacy practice and services utilizing telecommunications technology. As we discussed with telehealth and telemedicine, we can also contrast telepharmacy by the healthcare practitioner utilizing this treatment modality. We can see telepharmacy as the sole provision of licensed pharmacist providers and support staff working under their supervision (e.g., pharmacy technicians).[16] Lastly, ASHP's Practice Advancement Initiative (PAI) 2030 recommendations specifically addresses telepharmacy, stating that "virtual pharmacy services (e.g., telepharmacy) should be deployed to optimize operational and clinical services that extend patient care services and enhance continuity of care."[17]

Other Terminology

Synchronous Telehealth

Synchronous is defined as real-time telephonic or live audio and video interaction in the delivery of telehealth. In contemporary practice, this typically involves a patient using a smartphone, tablet, or computer to connect with their provider. In an alternate method, the synchronous care is provided by two healthcare professionals. For example, a nurse who is physically with the patient utilizes peripheral medical equipment (e.g., digital stethoscopes, otoscopes, ultrasounds) while consulting with the provider conducting the remote evaluation. Synchronous telehealth services are what most patients and practitioners are familiar with in the current pandemic environment. Most frequently, these services are delivered as a telephone call or video visit (via the Internet) between a healthcare practitioner and a patient, and they may include a caregiver or guardian such as a parent.

Asynchronous Telehealth

Asynchronous communication is defined as communication between parties that is not live (i.e., real time). Asynchronous telehealth can utilize tools such as short messaging service (SMS) messaging—commonly referred to as texting; electronic mail (email); voice messages; or use of digital patient portals. The ONC defines asynchronous telehealth as "store-and-forward videoconferencing," which is described as the transmission of a recorded health history or patient information to a provider.[6] The provider then reviews the stored data and makes diagnosis, treatment, and planning recommendations that are electronically delivered to either a referring provider, the patient, or the patient's caregiver. Online digital visits or patient check-in services via asynchronous technologies may also be utilized to evaluate whether or not an office visit is warranted. For a recent example of the utility of asynchronous telehealth, the Centers for Disease Control and Prevention (CDC) deployed V-safe, a smartphone-based application that uses SMS text messaging and web surveys to provide health check-ins after receiving the COVID-19 vaccine.[18]

Synchronous and asynchronous delivery of telehealth both reference the timing of the provision of healthcare services. An advantage of the synchronous approach is the efficiency gained by having the opportunity to seek additional information or data during the telehealth session, as well as providing clinical decisions or advice during the session. Conversely, efficiencies may nevertheless be obtained in asynchronous services when the telehealth episode does not require to-and-from interactions, especially when it does not rely on direct interaction with the patient throughout.[19]

Mobile Health (mHealth)

Mobile health (mHealth) is defined as healthcare and public health information that is provided through mobile devices. The information may include general educational information, targeted text messaging campaigns, and notifications about disease outbreaks.[6]

How is mHealth different from telehealth? The difference between mHealth and telehealth is that telehealth refers to all instances of healthcare via the use of modern technology, whereas mHealth refers to the concept of mobile health. Often, mHealth focuses on patient (or caregiver) self-care utilizing consumer technologies such as smartphone and tablet applications to capture their own health data. In its global survey of mHealth technologies, the World Health Organization (WHO) identifies 14 categories of mHealth services: health call centers, emergency toll-free telephone services, managing emergencies and disasters, mobile telemedicine, appointment reminders, community mobilization and health promotion, treatment compliance, mobile patient records, information access, patient monitoring, health surveys and data collection, surveillance, health awareness raising, and decision support systems. The survey findings state that the predominant form of mHealth today is characterized by small-scale pilot projects that address single issues in information sharing and access.[20]

eConsults

Electronic consultations (eConsults), also known as interprofessional consults, are communications between healthcare providers. Providers can use eConsults to get recommendations for complicated conditions from providers in other locations with additional expertise, for example, in specialty areas such as trauma or behavioral health.[21] Providers may interact with each other using a variety of telecommunications methods, such as electronic mail, SMS messaging, and phone or audio/video, and the eConsult may occur synchronously or asynchronously as warranted in the patient care scenario. Some of the benefits of eConsults in healthcare are increased care coordination, increased access to high-quality specialty care, accelerated consultation response time, reduction in unnecessary referrals, and transmission of clinical knowledge by interprofessional interactions.[21]

Web-Based Services

Web-based services are healthcare applications delivered via the Internet, accessed by patients via a web browser (or browser), which is application software for accessing the World Wide Web.[22-24] In contrast to web-based services, app-based services require a local application to be deployed and installed on a smartphone, tablet, or computer. From a deployment and availability perspective, web-based healthcare applications offer greater accessibility for both computer and mobile devices users. However, healthcare web-based services still require careful attention to local and federal regulatory requirements, as well as security. As an example of web-based services from a public health perspective, the ONC for Health Information Technology (HealthIT) maintains web-based applications that are interactive tools to visualize and analyze ONC's open-source data. For example, there is a web-based application that creates custom summaries of the latest national and state HealthIT data and statistics.[25]

CONCLUSION

This chapter introduced the term *telehealth* as the use of telecommunication technologies to deliver distanced healthcare. Additionally, we discussed the subsets of telehealth, which are telemedicine for the remote delivery of medicine and telepharmacy for the remote delivery of pharmacy services. Telehealth and the related services telemedicine and telepharmacy may be delivered synchronously, otherwise known as real time, using audio or audiovisual technologies; or delivered asynchronously using tools such as text message, email, and digital patient portals. RPM is an example of an asynchronous method of collecting remote patient clinical data for evaluation. Another example of asynchronous telecommunication between healthcare providers is eConsults, which is designed to gain rapid specialty advice and insight into patient conditions. Lastly, we also discussed how Telehealth can be deployed via application-based services (mHealth or mobile Health) and web-based services via the Internet. Both methods have the goal of addressing a patient's health status, but they are contrasted in different technological methods for delivery. Please keep these definitions in mind as you review subsequent chapters in this text and learn more about all aspects of telepharmacy.

REFERENCES

1. CMS Medicare Telehealth. **https://www.cms.gov/Medicare/Medicare-General-Information/Telehealth**. Accessed May 4, 2021.
2. AMA Telehealth quick guide | American Medical Association. **https://www.ama-assn.org/practice-management/digital/ama-telehealth-quick-guide**. Accessed May 4, 2021.
3. American Board of Telehealth. **https://www.americanboardoftelehealth.org**. Accessed May 4, 2021.
4. American Telemedicine Association. **https://www.americantelemed.org**. Accessed May 4, 2021.
5. National Consortium of Telehealth Resource Centers. **https://telehealthresourcecenter.org**. Accessed May 4, 2021.
6. Telemedicine and Telehealth | HealthIT.gov. **https://www.healthit.gov/topic/health-it-health-care-settings/telemedicine-and-telehealth**. Accessed May 4, 2021.
7. Telehealth Programs—Official website of the U.S. Health Resources. **https://www.hrsa.gov/rural-health/telehealth**. Accessed May 4, 2021.
8. Telehealth | HHS.gov. **https://www.hhs.gov/hipaa/for-professionals/faq/telehealth/index.html**. Accessed May 4, 2021.
9. What Is Telecommunications? Definition from Techopedia. **https://www.techopedia.com/definition/5570/telecommunications**. Accessed May 8, 2021.
10. Definition of Telecommunication by Merriam-Webster. **https://www.merriam-webster.com/dictionary/telecommunication**. Accessed May 8, 2021.
11. Using Telehealth to Expand Access to Essential Health Services. **https://www.cdc.gov/coronavirus/2019-ncov/hcp/telehealth.html**. Accessed May 8, 2021.
12. Telemedicine, Medicaid.gov. **https://www.medicaid.gov/medicaid/benefits/telemedicine/index.html**. Accessed May 8, 2021.
13. Telehealth resource center: Definitions | American Medical Association. **https://www.ama-assn.org/practice-management/digital/telehealth-resource-center-definitions**. Accessed May 8, 2021.
14. Model Pharmacy Act/Rules—NABP. **https://nabp.pharmacy/resources/model-pharmacy-act**. Accessed May 8, 2021.
15. ASHP statement on telepharmacy. *Am Health-Syst Pharm.* May 1, 2017; 74(9):e236-e241. **https://doi.org/10.2146/ajhp170039**. Accessed May 8, 2021.
16. Telehealth | American Pharmacists Association. **https://portal.pharmacist.com/Telehealth**. Accessed May 8, 2021.
17. American Society of Health-System Pharmacists (ASHP). Practice Advancement Initiative (PAI 2030). **https://www.ashp.org/Pharmacy-Practice/PAI**. Accessed May 8, 2021.
18. V-safe After Vaccination Health Checker | CDC. **https://www.cdc.gov/coronavirus/2019-ncov/vaccines/safety/vsafe.html**. Accessed May 8, 2021.
19. Wilson LS, Maeder AJ. Recent directions in telemedicine: Review of trends in research and practice. *Healthc Inform Res*. 2015;21(4):213-222. doi:10.4258/hir.2015.21.4.213.
20. mhealth New horizons for health through mobile technologies. World Health Organization (WHO). **https://www.who.int/goe/publications/goe_mhealth_web.pdf**. Accessed May 8, 2021.
21. E-consults | Telehealth.HHS.gov. **https://telehealth.hhs.gov/providers/telehealth-for-emergency-departments/e-consults**. Accessed May 9, 2021.
22. Wikipedia contributors. World Wide Web. Wikipedia, The Free Encyclopedia. May 4, 2021, 14:09 UTC. **https://en.wikipedia.org/w/index.php?title=World_Wide_Web&oldid=1021398347**. Accessed May 9, 2021.
23. Wikipedia contributors. Web browser. Wikipedia, The Free Encyclopedia. May 9, 2021, 01:13 UTC. **https://en.wikipedia.org/w/index.php?title=Web_browser&oldid=1022189630**. Accessed May 9, 2021.
24. Web-based vs App-Based—Telehealth Features Series | Healthcare IT Today. **https://www.healthcareittoday.com/2020/07/23/web-based-vs-app-based-telehealth-features-series**. Accessed May 9, 2021.
25. Health IT Apps. Healthit.gov. **https://dashboard.healthit.gov/apps/apps.php**. Accessed May 9, 2021.

CHAPTER 3 Integration of Telehealth into Contemporary Pharmacy Practice

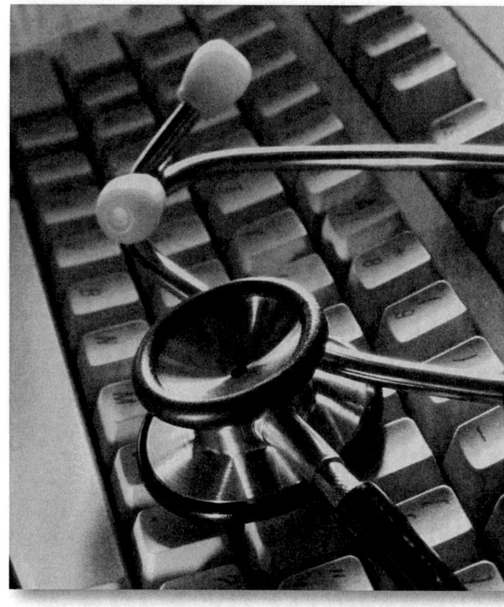

Pharmacists have been providing telehealth services for more than 20 years. As the use of the World Wide Web increased in the early 2000s, medication therapy management (MTM) platforms were developed in order to allow pharmacists to complete comprehensive medication reviews and targeted medication interventions for patients as a part of Medicare and some state Medicaid MTM programs. Health-system pharmacists have provided comprehensive medication management and disease state management services via telehealth pharmacy practice (primarily telephone visits) for much longer.

The COVID-19 epidemic accelerated the use of telehealth by health systems for various visits that would otherwise have been in person. Previously, many of these visits were conducted in person to allow the provider to use physical examination as part of the visit. Most pharmacist visits were conducted in person also because prior to the pandemic, telehealth visits were not reimbursed by insurance companies to a large extent. COVID-19 forced providers to become creative in the use of physical examination via telehealth. It also allowed a mechanism for reimbursement for these types of visits, making them more financially viable.

During the COVID-19 pandemic, Medicare temporarily lifted several restrictions on the types of services that were reimbursed when conducted via telehealth. Medicare also relaxed Health Insurance Portability and Accountability Act (HIPAA) privacy laws that allow the use of smartphones for telehealth visits. They allowed video-conferencing platforms such as Zoom and messaging services like WhatsApp to be used for telehealth visits. Regulations were also relaxed to allow for the provision of care across state lines in 48 states.[1]

An analysis conducted by Brigham Health in Boston estimated that 50% of visits could be conducted virtually, as they did not require physical examination or testing in order to establish a diagnosis and treatment plan. Because many of the medication management services provided by pharmacists do not require a physical exam, they are ideal candidates for remote care. Tele-video visits with high-quality video may be preferred to audio-only visits by some pharmacists and patients because it allows the pharmacist to instruct on the administration of various medication delivery devices and to see the patient's medication bottles and home environment, which can give the pharmacist valuable information when formulating their assessment and plan.[2,3]

COMPARISON OF PLATFORMS

Many methods can be used to provide pharmacy telehealth services, including video, secure texting, telephone or Internet-audio, and remote monitoring systems (see **Table 3.1** for examples of platforms). Each of these methods has benefits and drawbacks. Within

DOI 10.37573/9781585286928.003

each of these methods, there are many options to choose from, and the market is evolving rapidly in order to keep up with the growing pace of telehealth utilization.

Some of these platforms integrate directly into the electronic health record, while others do not. For example, Zoom provides a way to conduct HIPAA-compliant video calls with patients, but it does not have capability for scheduling or billing, which may be done separately within the electronic health records (EHRs).

Some systems require a patient to download an app onto their device in order to participate in the visit, while others only require a camera, microphone, and Internet connection. One must consider both the ease of use for the consumer and the training required for the healthcare professional who provides the service. Some platforms provide IT support, while others require more support from the healthcare setting's IT department.[4] (For more information, refer to Section 2: Telehealth Pharmacy Practice Workflows.)

Table 3.1. Examples of Telehealth Platforms[5-10]

Mode	Platform	Characteristics
Video	Zoom	Healthcare Zoom requires a paid subscription HIPAA compliant Integrates within some EHRs Closed captioning available Sessions can be recorded onto a desktop hard drive Passcodes and waiting rooms provide security
	Doximity	Free and paid subscription options available No recording capability No downloads or sign-on required for patients Video or audio-only calls available Electronic medical record (EMR) integration available with paid option
	OhMD	No downloads or sign-on required for patients EMR integration available
	doxy.me	Free and paid options available Can schedule and bill for appointments within the platform with the paid version
	Mend	Requires a paid subscription Can integrate with EHR Allows for scheduling and billing
	EVisit	Requires a paid subscription; integrates with some EHRs, allows for scheduling and billing
Texting	OhMD	HIPAA compliant Can use practice phone number Conversations can be saved in the EHR through EHR integration options
Secure patient messaging	Many EHR platforms	Requires sign-in Typically asynchronous communication
Remote patient monitoring (RPM)	DexCom ResMed Medtronic Phillips Healthcare Optimize Health	Weight, blood pressure, heart rate, pulse oximetry, blood glucose, medication adherence, behavioral health surveys

Preferred Platforms for Different Types of Healthcare Settings

There are many aspects to consider when determining the "best" platform for a telehealth pharmacy practice encounter. Does the practice site already have a functioning EHR and practice management system? If so, one may only need to add a video platform with which to provide telehealth. If the practice site does not have an EHR or practice management system, one might consider purchasing a system that integrates telehealth visits within the platform but also gives all of the other features that are important to running a successful ambulatory practice, such as documentation, scheduling, and billing.

Privacy and Security of Telehealth Visits

Before beginning a discussion of privacy and security during pharmacy telehealth visits, it is important to define these terms. *Security* is protection against the unauthorized access of data, whereas *privacy* relates to *who* has access to specific data. These terms can be difficult to define, and the two overlap.[11,12]

Privacy and security of health information during telehealth encounters can be addressed in several ways. Digital communication between providers and patients is often encrypted to reduce the risk of unauthorized access to data. Patients are frequently required to sign a consent before participating in telehealth, acknowledging how their digital information may be used. However, patients often do not read or understand privacy policies. Health information can be available through multiple methods, including the use of apps for remote patient monitoring or telehealth encounters.[13]

Skype, FaceTime, Facebook Messenger Video, Google Hangouts Video, and some Zoom applications may not meet all of the requirements of HIPAA. During the COVID-19 pandemic, the Department of Health and Human Services (DHS) has not fully enforced these requirements, while healthcare professionals are working to provide telehealth services to an increasing number of patients. However, when the public health emergency ends, providers will need to transition to a HIPAA-compliant telehealth platform. Public-facing platforms are never acceptable for providing telehealth. Those providers who choose to use those platforms (such as TikTok, Facebook Live, and Twitch) may be subject to enforcement actions for violations of HIPAA.[14]

BENEFITS OF TELEHEALTH PHARMACY PRACTICE

There are many benefits to telehealth pharmacy practice visits that can help the pharmacist to provide better care for patients. These benefits may include the following:

1. The pharmacist is able to see the patient's home environment. Where does the patient store their medications? Are there safety concerns? Who else lives in their home who would never accompany them to their in-person appointments but may play a role in the patient's ability to manage their medications?[3]
2. The patient is less likely to miss their appointment. One clinician reported that their no-show rate was less than 10%, which is lower than in-person visits. Some of these patients have missed their in-person appointments in the past due to transportation, work, or child care challenges. Telehealth is an easier option for those patients.[15]
3. The patient may be more comfortable in their own environment. The process of traveling to a clinic, checking in, and being in an unfamiliar exam room surrounded by medical equipment causes anxiety for some patients. The ability to conduct a visit with a healthcare provider within the comfort of their own home may result in improved interaction between the patient and provider.[16]

BARRIERS TO TELEHEALTH

There are many barriers to wider implementation of telehealth encounters. These barriers may include the following:

- *Telehealth is viewed as impersonal.* A subset of patients and providers view telehealth visits as more impersonal and disconnected when compared to in-person interactions. This can be related to blurry video images, audio or video lag time, and an inability to clearly see the other's nonverbal communication, such as facial expressions, gestures, and body language.
- *Technology poses challenges.* There may be insufficient Wifi or cell signal strength in the patient's home for real-time video. The resolution of the video may make it difficult to see each other clearly. The patient may not have a smartphone and thus will be unable to send photos of derm concerns, surgical sites, medication bottles, and so on, to the clinician. A recent Kaiser Family Foundation poll found that only 68% of older adults have a way to engage in video visits from home using a computer, tablet, or smartphone with adequate Internet access. The patient may also lack the technological literacy to utilize the telehealth platform to its fullest potential.[17-19]
- *Distractions may emerge.* If conducting telehealth via the phone, the patient may become distracted by other things or people in their home and not give the provider their undivided attention.

The National Telehealth Technology Assessment Resource Center gives some helpful tips for making the most of a telehealth visit, including lighting, camera position, and how to focus on objects of interest to the clinician, such as skin lesions or medication bottles.[20]

Technology Literacy and Access

The patient's ability to successfully use telehealth platforms has a direct impact on the ability of the healthcare professional to impact health outcomes and to identify and resolve medication-related problems. Many patients, particularly the elderly, have challenges with accessing the platforms used for telehealth. They may not have experience with downloading applications, using a webcam, and adjusting audio to allow for optimal communication during telehealth visits. During pandemics such as COVID-19, where younger family members or neighbors are not able to help due to social distancing, healthcare organizations may find that these visits cannot meet their goals because of the time that it takes to troubleshoot technical issues during the visit. The Vanderbilt University Health System solves these challenges by utilizing medical student volunteers to connect with patients prior to their scheduled telehealth visits to set up and test the telehealth platform.[21,22]

Even when the technology is tested ahead of time, however, there can still be challenges during the visit. Unanticipated barriers may arise at any point during scheduled telehealth pharmacy practice visits within a large health system. Although the test was successful prior to the visit, a lack of adequate bandwidth resulted in the provider and patient being unable to use video during the visit.

Access to Technology Resources

In addition to the lack of technology literacy, lack of access to hardware, software, and reliable broadband services results in challenges when conducting telehealth visits. This is typically thought of as a rural challenge, but it can also occur in urban and suburban areas. Smartphones can be utilized for telehealth visits, but many patients own cellular phones that are not capable of real-time video interaction. Both patients and providers may find that using a bigger screen on a desktop computer, laptop computer, or tablet may provide for a better video experience. If the patient does not have sufficient Internet speed in their home, due to either cost constraints or lack of adequate broadband connection, video and audio can break up, impacting the ability of the patient and provider to communicate effectively.

For patients with limited English proficiency who require interpreter services, telehealth visits can present an additional challenge. Many telehealth platforms were not designed to easily integrate a medical interpreter into the visit. One health system in California was able to successfully integrate medical interpreters into video visits using both the Epic MyChart and Zoom platforms by developing a workflow that allowed the provider to schedule an interpreter via the electronic medical record (EMR) and allowed the interpreter to join an existing encounter without compromising privacy and security concerns. The Health Resource Services Administration (HRSA), a division of Health and Human Services, offers tips for how to effectively provide telehealth to patients with limited English proficiency.[23-25]

Billing for Pharmacy Telehealth Services

Billing for ambulatory pharmacist services has always been a challenge and often must be pieced together using various methods depending on the setting and patient population. This is no difference when discussing pharmacist billing for telehealth services. Hospitals may bill as the originating site of care when the patient is located at homes through Medicare Part A. Medicare Part B also pays for video and telephone E &M services and education services. Medicare telehealth services are paid at the same rate as visits occurring in the office. Medicare also pays for virtual check-ins via telephone discussions, secure patient portal, or secure video. These can be synchronous or asynchronous. E-visits are non-face-to-face visits conducted through a patient portal. Medicare will reimburse for these visits. Medicare maintains a list of services for which providers may bill for telehealth services on their website. Some of these services are temporary additions, introduced during the public health emergency, and some are permanent inclusions.[26]

WHAT DOES THIS MEAN FOR PHARMACISTS?

Pharmacists can bill for telehealth services "incident-to" a Medicare-recognized provider (physician). Services that have required direct supervision in which the physician is present in the same office suite are now waived as well; this supervision can be provided remotely. For quite some time now, pharmacists have been providing and have been paid for medication therapy management (MTM), including comprehensive medication reviews (CMRs) and targeted medication reviews for patients with Medicare Part D. This is the most common method for paying pharmacists for providing telehealth services. These services are generally paid for by the pharmacy benefit manager (PBM) or a third-party company that contracts with the PBM. This system has not changed in the face of the public health emergency.[27]

Pharmacists have also participated as part of the interprofessional clinic team in providing transitional care management (TCM) and chronic care management (CCM) services via telehealth, and the provision of and reimbursement for these services has not changed during the pandemic. (For additional information, see Section 3: Exploring Revenue Opportunities with Telehealth for Pharmacists.)

Through familiarity with the basic terminology, history, and infrastructure of telehealth, pharmacists will be prepared to successfully incorporate this growing healthcare service into their future practices. The following chapters will explore in greater detail the specifics of clinical workflows, billing, metrics, and educational opportunities for learners, which are all essential elements in building a successful and integrated telehealth practice model.

REFERENCES

1. Van Beusekom M. In Pandemic, Many Seeing Upside of Telemedicine. University of Minnesota Center for Infectious Disease Research and Policy. **https://www.cidrap.umn.edu/news-perspective/2020/05/pandemic-many-seeing-upsides-telemedicine**. Published May 21, 2020. Accessed February 28, 2021.
2. Licurse A. Fanning K. Laskowski K. Landman A. Balancing Virtual and In-Person Health Care. *Harv Bus Rev*. **https://hbr.org/2020/11/balancing-virtual-and-in-person-health-care**. Published November 17, 2020. Accessed February 28, 2021.
3. Traynor K. Pharmacists Turn to Telehealth to Meet Patients' Needs. American Society of Health-System Pharmacists. **https://www.ashp.org/News/2020/07/29/Pharmacists-Turn-to-Telehealth-to-Meet-Patients-Needs?loginreturnUrl=SSOCheckOnly**. Published July 29, 2020. Accessed February 28, 2021.
4. Riley E. Telemedicine Platform Options and How to Choose the Best One for Your Practice. GoodRx. **https://www.goodrx.com/blog/telemedicine-platform-practice-provider-options-how-to-choose**. Published April 17, 2020. Accessed February 15, 2021.
5. Optimize Health Remote Patient Monitoring Software Platform. **https://www.optimize.health/remote-patient-monitoring-and-patient-engagement-platform**. Accessed October 24, 2021.
6. Zoom for Healthcare. **https://zoom.us/healthcare**. Accessed February 15, 2021.
7. Doximity. **https://www.doximity.com/dialer**. Accessed February 15, 2021.
8. OhMD. **https://www.ohmd.com/patient-communication**. Accessed February 15, 2021.
9. Centers for Disease Control and Prevention. Using Telehealth to Expand Access to Essential Health Services during the COVID-19 Pandemic. **https://www.cdc.gov/coronavirus/2019-ncov/hcp/telehealth.html**. Updated June 10, 2020. Accessed February 15, 2021.
10. Dolan S. The Technology, Devices, and Benefits of Remote Patient Monitoring in the Healthcare Industry. Business Insider. **https://www.businessinsider.com/remote-patient-monitoring-industry-explained**. Published March 10, 2021. Accessed May 3, 2021.
11. Hiv.gov. The Difference between Security and Privacy and Why It Matters to Your Program. **https://www.hiv.gov/blog/difference-between-security-and-privacy-and-why-it-matters-your-program#:~:text=What%20is%20the%20Difference%20between,the%20safeguarding%20of%20user%20identity.&text=Security%20refers%20to%20protection%20against,who%20can%20access%20the%20information**. Published April 26, 2018. Accessed February 15, 2021.
12. Office for Civil Rights. Summary of the HIPAA Security Rule. **https://www.hhs.gov/hipaa/for-professionals/security/laws-regulations/index.html**. Updated July 26, 2013. Accessed February 15, 2021.
13. Hall JL, McGraw D. For telehealth to succeed, privacy and security risks must be assessed and addressed. *Health Affairs*. 2014;33(2):216-221.
14. Office for Civil Rights. Notification of Enforcement Discretion for Telehealth Remote Communications during the COVID-19 Pandemic. **https://www.hhs.gov/hipaa/for-professionals/special-topics/emergency-preparedness/notification-enforcement-discretion-telehealth/index.html**. Updated January 20, 2021. Accessed February 15, 2021.
15. Van Beusekom M. COVID-19 Reveals Telehealth Barriers, Solutions. **https://www.cidrap.umn.edu/news-perspective/2020/05/covid-19-reveals-telehealth-barriers-solutions**. Published May 22, 2020. Accessed February 28, 2021.
16. Powell RE, Henstenburg JM, Cooper G, et al. Patient perceptions of telehealth primary care video visits. *Ann Fam Med*. 2017;15(3):225-229.
17. Cubanski J. Possibilities and Limits of Telehealth for Older Adults during the COVID-19 Emergency. **https://www.kff.org/policy-watch/possibilities-and-limits-of-telehealth-for-older-adults-during-the-covid-19-emergency**. Published April 13, 2020. Accessed February 15, 2021.
18. International Technology and Engineering Educators Association. Technologically Literate Citizens. **https://www.iteea.org/48897.aspx#:~:text=The%20term%20%E2%80%9Ctechnological%20literacy%E2%80%9D%20refers,turn%20how%20society%20shapes%20it**. Accessed April 25, 2021.
19. Blandford A, Wesson J, Amalberti R, et al. Opportunities and challenges for telehealth within, and beyond, a pandemic. *The Lancet Global Health*. 2020;8(11):E1364-E1365.
20. National Telehealth and Technology Resource Center. Video Platforms: Customer Point of View. **https://telehealthtechnology.org/toolkit/customer-point-of-view**. Accessed May 3, 2021.
21. Triana AJ, Gusdorf RE, Shah KP, Horst SN. Technology literacy as a barrier to telehealth during COVID-19. *Telemedicine and E-health*. 2020;26(9):1118-1119.

22. Clendening J. VUSM Students Help Patients, Clinicians with Telehealth. **https://news.vumc.org/2020/04/23/vusm-students-help-patients-clinicians-with-telehealth**. Published April 23, 2020. Accessed May 3, 2021.
23. Quinlan K. Remote Interpreters Are Critical in the Shift to Telehealth. **https://multilingual.com/remote-interpreters-are-critical-in-the-shift-to-telehealth**. Published November 4, 2020. Accessed February 15, 2021.
24. Hsu M. Integration of Interpreting Services into Video Visit Program Shows Commitment to Health Equity, Diversity, and Inclusion. **https://health.ucdavis.edu/health-news/newsroom/integration-of-interpreting-services-into-video-visit-program-shows-commitment-to-health-equity-diversity-and-inclusion/2020/05**. Published May 12, 2020. Accessed February 15, 2021.
25. Improving Access to Telehealth. **https://telehealth.hhs.gov/providers/increasing-telehealth-equity-and-access/improving-access-to-telehealth**. Updated February 9, 2021. Accessed February 15, 2021.
26. Billing for Telehealth during COVID-19. **https://telehealth.hhs.gov/providers/billing-and-reimbursement**. Accessed February 15, 2021.
27. Issue Brief: COVID-19 and Telehealth Changes. **https://www.ashp.org/Advocacy-and-Issues/Key-Issues/Other-Issues/Issue-Brief-COVID-19?loginreturnUrl=SSOCheckOnly**. Published April 9, 2020. Accessed February 15, 2021.

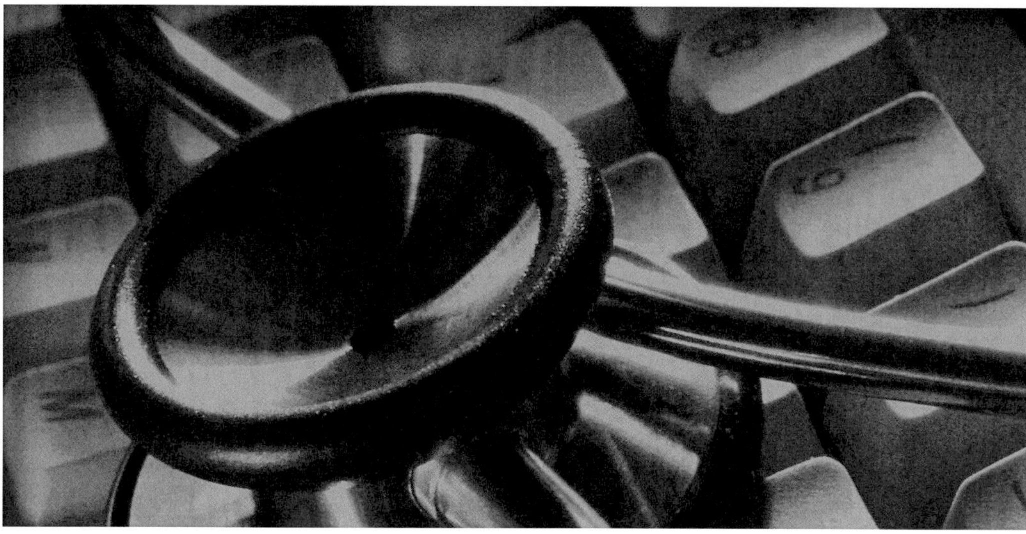

SECTION 2
Telehealth Pharmacy Practice Workflows

Felix K. Yam, Megan Dorrell, Heather Jones, and M. Shawn McFarland

CHAPTER 4 Foundational Steps for Designing Telehealth Pharmacy Practice Care Models

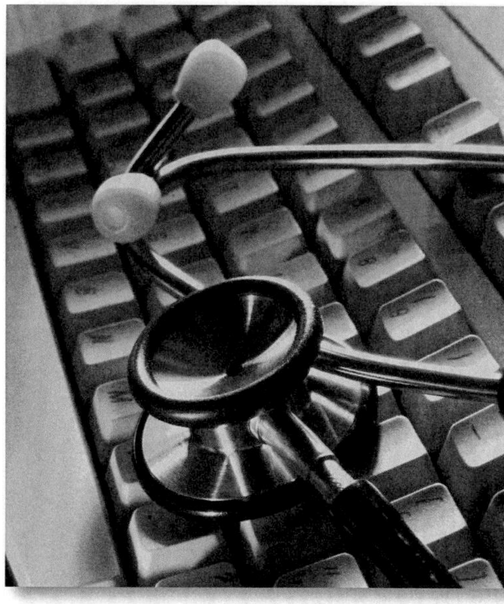

Once the foundations for telehealth services have been established in your institution, successful implementation of telehealth pharmacy practice will require an effective and efficient workflow. Your team must be prepared to utilize telehealth technologies, train medical staff and patients, conduct the visit, perform administrative functions (e.g., electronically rooming patients, setting up appointments), implement quality assessments, and establish billing procedures. Furthermore, these new practices need to be incorporated into the clinics' existing workflow if a hybrid of telehealth and in-person patient care visits is developed.

Many of the activities associated with telehealth and in-person clinical encounters will be similar, but the delivery of telehealth pharmacy practice services will present unique opportunities and challenges. These changes will require the development of new workflows. This chapter explores necessary considerations when developing workflows for telehealth pharmacy practice services. Moreover, we will address specific barriers to successful implementation and recommend strategies to overcome these barriers.

PREPARING FOR TELEHEALTH PHARMACY PRACTICE APPOINTMENTS

Workflow Mapping

The implementation of telehealth may present many changes to your existing workflow. Prior to implementing telehealth, it is important to have a good understanding of the current clinic workflow. This will help identify necessary modifications to existing workflow to accommodate and integrate telehealth pharmacy practice visits. A visual representation of your clinic workflow is helpful to identify the entire work process before, during, and after the appointment. Tasks such as patient registration, scheduling, rooming, performing vitals, patient education, and follow-up scheduling need to be adapted to accommodate a remote environment. Workflow varies widely among institutions and must be customized to each individual institution and organization. Basic steps to creating a workflow diagram are listed in **Table 4.1**.

DOI 10.37573/9781585286928.004

Table 4.1. Basic Steps to Creating Workflow[1]

1. Clarify the purpose or outcome of the process.
2. Identify a clear start and end point for the process.
3. List or draw out the tasks and decision points within the process and put them in order.
4. Define and note which role completes each step.
5. Identify and name the process.

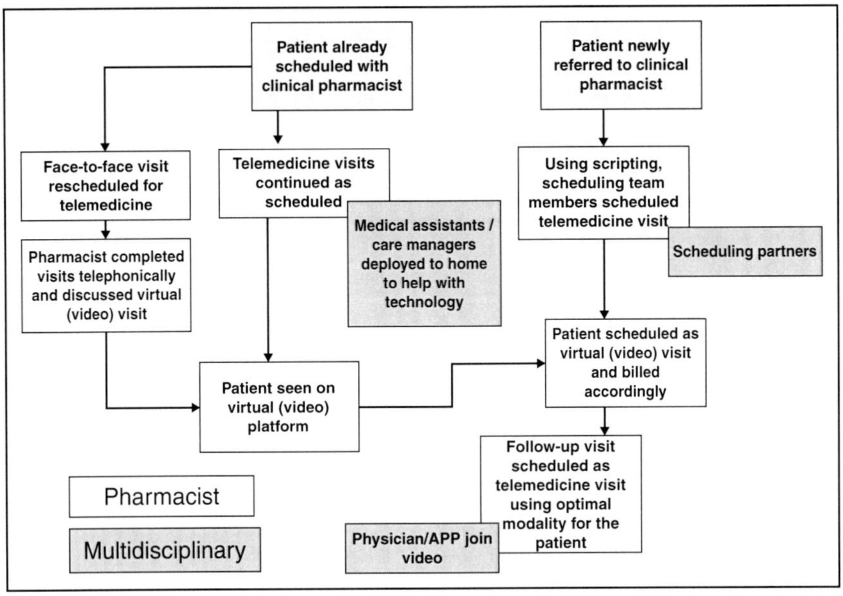

Figure 4.1. Example for visual workflow for telehealth pharmacy practice: care flow for multidisciplinary intersection points

Source: DeRemer CE, Reiter J, Olson JL. Transitioning ambulatory care pharmacy services to telemedicine while maintaining multidisciplinary collaborations. *Am J Health-Syst Pharm*. 2021;78(5):371-375. Permission from Oxford University Press.

Important elements of workflow include the consideration of physical and/or mental tasks, role delineation, work processes, and communication with other members of the team or external organizations. Developing a workflow map that shows a picture of these steps can be helpful in standardizing processes and identifying where gaps may exist (**Figure 4.1**). Workflow tasks can be sequential or simultaneous and should be customized to your clinic. Sequential tasks occur in a stepwise fashion, whereas simultaneous tasks rely on coordination of staff to perform tasks at the same time.

In addition to mapping the process for patient encounters, it is important to clearly identify who performs each task. Most ambulatory care clinics rely on multiple disciplines for a variety of tasks. Telehealth pharmacy services may bring additional challenges when team members are working remotely. Additional methods for communication between team members may be needed to ensure that these tasks are completed. Synchronization of these tasks in a remote environment will require careful coordination. **Table 4.2** lists key questions to consider with workflow mapping, and **Table 4.3** lists examples of clinic-level workflows.

Table 4.2. Key Questions to Consider in Workflow Mapping for Telehealth[2,3]

• How will patients be informed of the availability of telehealth services?
• What technology requirements will be needed for providers and patients?
• What staff will be involved in scheduling telehealth appointments and coordinating with remote specialists?
• How will staff manage referrals?
• On the day of the telehealth encounter, who will educate/train the patient?
• Who is responsible for coordinating patient follow-up?
• For remote patient monitoring, how will staff receive data?
• How will you handle billing?

Table 4.3. Example of Clinic Workflows for Telehealth

• Answering phones	• Reporting diagnostic test results
• Appointment system	• Ordering medications
• Messaging	• Referrals
• Scheduling procedures	• Follow-up
• Ordering diagnostics/labs	

Clinic-level workflows are important for ensuring smooth operations between clinic staff, provider, pharmacist, and patients. In addition to clinic-level workflows, interorganizational workflows must also be considered. For example, workflow between the pharmacist, the patient's primary care provider, specialty providers, and community pharmacy also needs to be considered. The process for communication with external organizations may not differ from traditional visits, but considerations may need to be made if clinic personnel are working remotely. One strategy to create your workflows is to visualize the process into three separate phases: pre-visit, telehealth visit, and post-visit. Throughout each of these steps, care should be taken to consider the flow of communication.

Pre-visit Workflow

In the pre-visit phase, your process should include delegation of personnel that will contact the patient and ensure the patient is prepared for and has consented to the telehealth visit. Institutions may designate clinical or nonclinical staff for this task. In some instances, call centers may be utilized to perform initial patient contact. Where call centers or nonclinical staff are utilized, clear instructions must be provided on what to communicate to patients (e.g., purpose of visit, information requirements, and expectations for technology). A designated person should also evaluate what clinical data (e.g., vitals, laboratory measurements) are needed for the encounter and determine how this information will be provided by the patient and made available to the provider. Designated staff will need to perform a technology assessment to determine if the patient is able to provide the necessary clinical data prior to or during the remote patient encounter.

Patients should be told what to expect from the encounter and what services will be provided. Confirmation of these assessments then needs to be documented, with communication back to the responsible party conducting the telehealth pharmacy practice visit. Daily staff huddles with providers and pharmacist can be useful to communicate this information. In remote settings, teleconferencing can be utilized to ensure appropriate information is communicated to all responsible and participating parties.

Telehealth Visit

Policies and procedures should be developed to guide the telehealth pharmacy practice visit. All parties, including the patient, need to be trained on the platform being used. Accommodations may be needed for certain patient populations during the encounter. Workflows should consider the need for medical interpreter and/or other means of communication for those with disabilities (e.g., visual, hearing, or cognitive). Integrating these needs during the telehealth visit may require careful coordination with external organizations and interface capabilities with your clinics' telehealth technologies.

As part of the telehealth visit, patients may need to perform self-monitoring clinical assessments (e.g., blood glucose, blood pressure, pulse, weight). These measurements may be self-reported or transmitted electronically if technology permits. If self-reported, the pharmacist conducting telehealth pharmacy visits should ensure measurements are accurately recorded into the medical record in the proper locations. Permission to access documentation may be needed from the institution, so evaluation of this access point has to be considered prior to conducting patient encounters. Where clinical data can be transmitted electronically (e.g., connected to smart devices), the data should be summarized and documented in the patient's medical record prior to the telehealth visit so that the information is readily available during the encounter.

Post-visit Workflow

The post-visit phase includes everything that occurs once the pharmacist has evaluated the patient. This includes assessment of the patient's problems and development of a plan for the patient, as well as communication and education of the plan to the patient and provider. Once the plan is communicated, the encounter must be documented and any changes to the patient care plan need to be transmitted. For example, new prescriptions will need to be transmitted to the patient's pharmacy electronically. Referrals will need to be entered into the system. The type of follow-up should be determined (e.g., face-to-face or telehealth) and should be scheduled. Workflow mapping can help determine who is responsible for these tasks and how they will get done.

In collaborative practice models where pharmacists are working with other healthcare providers, additional considerations should ensure that recommendations are communicated and that the plan of care is executed. Most electronic health records should have provisions for pharmacists to enter orders that are then cosigned by physicians. Appropriate alerts and flags need to be in place to ensure timely execution of these clinical orders. Staff huddles or teleconferencing to review patient encounters are useful to ensure appropriate follow-up of patient care plans.

CONDUCTING A TELEHEALTH PHARMACY PRACTICE APPOINTMENT

While telehealth might be new to the reader's practice, the skills needed to be successful in telehealth mirror the skills needed for successful clinical pharmacist care while face-to-face. Patient connections and relationship building through use of motivational interviewing, patient and medication assessment with optimization of therapies with evidence, and enhancement of patient education remain central to the telehealth patient care experience. Let's take a look at some of the essential components of the telehealth pharmacy practice appointments utilizing the considerations we have discussed.

Pre-visit Assessment

Prior to the start of a telehealth pharmacy practice appointment, an assessment should be completed to see if the patient is a good candidate for telehealth. During the scheduling or identification process, the patient's expectation for the appointment can be defined, assessment of the patient's understanding of health technology can be completed, and a decision can be made on a delivery method for the telehealth pharmacy practice experience. Another approach is to predefine patient visit types that would benefit from the telehealth pharmacy practice model prior to scheduling. For example, the reader could define that all insulin titration appointments could be offered as a telehealth pharmacy practice appointment. If possible, you can collaborate with clinic administration to identify resources within your network to allow for this administrative work to be completed by clinic support staff. If a medical assistant, pharmacy technician, or scheduling support individual is not available, consider using students and other learners to support workflow processes, keeping in consideration time when they will not be available (e.g., holidays, school breaks).

An important organizational step is to set the expectation for reminder calls or electronic reminder processes to contact the patient as to when and how to access the appointment platform. This step is especially important if the patient is used to seeing their pharmacist face-to-face in their provider's office. If the patient is remaining at home, they should be reminded to remain home. If the patient is going to a satellite medical office, they should be informed of the address, as well as, if it is their first visit, information specific to the location that may be different from their home clinic experience. If not previously decided upon, this would be the time to decide if the visit will be a telephonic appointment or a tele-video, including which platform will be used if your practice allows for multiple options. Patients should also be educated on how to join in the experience, who to expect to interact with, and what they should have near them during the appointment. Prepping patients to have medication vials, medication lists, blood glucose monitor or logs, blood pressure monitor or logs, and any other logs or assessment tools nearby avoids delays during the appointment. If reminder processes are being completed in the days prior to the appointment, the patient can also be instructed to complete necessary lab work to help with assessment during the appointment.

On the day of the visit, it may be important to have the patient checked in per normal processes. This check-in experience may vary based on expectations from the practice site. When a patient comes onsite to meet with a pharmacist, the front desk may verify changes in personal information and insurance, and check the patient in to meet the requirements in your electronic medical record (EMR). When this physical front desk is removed, what processes will be put in place to ensure that these activities are completed with the use of support staff, as available? If the telehealth pharmacy practice experience has the patient coming into a satellite location, that staff needs to be aware of the need to check in pharmacy clinic patients. Increased communication and planning around the check-in experience is an important workflow step to consider.

Conducting the Telehealth Pharmacy Practice Encounter

When it is time to start the telehealth pharmacy practice encounter, as with a face-to-face visit, the rooming of a patient begins the experience. Rooming of a patient may vary based on the setting, but traditional activities include bringing the patient back into a patient care space, obtaining vitals and other physical assessments, completing screenings, and updating the patient's medical record. In current workflow, this may be done by support individuals, pharmacy student or pharmacy resident, or the pharmacist completing that appointment. A workflow plan for these activities in telehealth is needed with higher attention paid to the regulatory requirements for these experiences, while providing the care via telehealth. For example, which vitals can be entered as patient self-reported?

If the patient is going into another medical facility to meet with the pharmacist through facility-based telehealth, the clinic support staff at the site can aid in this rooming. Deciding on workflow for vitals, EMR updates, and medication reviews is important. Establishing what point-of-care testing or lab facilities are onsite can help in the flow of the patient experience.

The telehealth pharmacy practice experience where the patient is at home leads to increased complexity. Patients may or may not have supplies at home to obtain vitals such as blood pressure, weight, or oxygen saturation. Adding to the complexity is how you are able to add vitals to the patient's medical record. It is key that you understand what can be added to a patient's medical record via self-reporting home vitals and what needs to be facility obtained. For example, during the COVID-19 pandemic, patient's blood pressure results for controlling high blood pressure or comprehensive diabetes care measure for Healthcare Effectiveness Data and Information Set (HEDIS) have not been allowed to be self-reported.[4] Another consideration for patient-reported vitals is recording the date and time of when the vital was obtained. If the patient provided a weight, was that obtained at the start of the appointment or the last time they checked, which may have been weeks ago? Including this date with the reporting may aid in finding patterns and allow for proper assessment. As telehealth rapidly expands, there is opportunity for more EMRs to have a designation between patient-provided and facility-obtained vitals. With the addition of this option, the complexity of reporting vitals should diminish. Another growth opportunity for consideration in this space is the use of remote patient monitoring as addressed in previous chapters.

Patient Assessment during Encounter

Providing patient and medication use assessment during telehealth pharmacy practice may vary based on the experience selected. If the appointment is provided via a tele-video experience, you should ensure that you are able to see the patient clearly to be able to assess nonverbal cues. With telephone-based telehealth, the added complexity of not viewing the patient needs to be considered. If the lack of nonverbal cues may impact the assessment, the choice may be made to limit the types of experiences that occur over the phone, such as selecting quick check-in-type discussions versus complete appointments. It may also be decided that complex new information discussions, such as starting insulin therapy for the first time, occur over tele-video or face-to-face if patient safety might be at risk without an expanded assessment of understanding.

Patient Education Delivery

Patient education comes in many forms, all of which need to be considered in telehealth workflows. In face-to-face encounters, disease state and general medication-related education may have been provided via patient-facing handouts or booklets. The reader may have also relied on sharing video or websites with patients while face-to-face together. Now that the patient and the pharmacist are in a different location, it is still feasible to provide this same level of education, but workflow adjustments will be needed. Ideally, developing a process to share materials with patients in real time should be optimized. Some EMRs allow for sharing PDF documents directly with patients through their patient portal. If PDFs are not available, patient education items may need to be mailed to the patient's house, which involves preplanning, post-appointment reliable execution, and time to allow for delivery. A secure email may also be a possible route to explore. Working with the information technology (IT) department to discover options is recommended. For videos or other online options, it may be possible to send them to the patient for them to watch, with you listening in. A better option may be to enable the patient to share your screen, which is available on some tele-video platforms. With this option, it is vital that you clear your screen of all other items not related to the care of the current patient.

Verbal patient education can continue similarly to verbal education in a face-to-face environment. Assessment of a patient's understanding of patient education, changes in therapy plans and medications, and other provided information may need to be expanded in telehealth. With a tele-video visit, you may find that your normal assessment of nonverbal cues and your normal practice of motivation interviewing fit the patient care experience. However, even with a video visit, a different approach to education may be needed inasmuch as you are in a different location than the patient. As above, with a telephone visit, you might find that the lack of nonverbal cues is a barrier that may lead you to select which activities to provide via telephone assessment and which activities to shift to tele-video or face-to-face visit. For example, when starting a new inhaler for a patient with a history of previously poor inhaler technique, you could decide that a visit should occur in person or at least in a two-way tele-video visit.

After completion of an appointment, patients may have an expectation of a physical updated medication list or written instructions for medication or care plan changes. Encouraging the use of patient portals should be a priority if they are available in your EMR. For patients without access to a patient portal, or for those who prefer paper copies of information, a copy of select informational items can be mailed. It is important that mailing occurs quickly after the appointment so as not to delay patient changes. Mailing the patient information may also add a level of complexity if the pharmacist is providing care out of their home. It may be best to consider pulling resources and having a contact physically onsite in the clinic that can print and mail materials.

Post-visit Planning

While patient assessment should be done prior to the appointment for appropriateness of telehealth pharmacy practice delivery of care, it should continue throughout the patient's care. The reader should assess if the current appointment was successful in meeting the patient's and the healthcare team's goals. If it was not, assessment should be made as to how to best deliver the next appointment.

Telehealth pharmacy practice models may also cause you to assess how you provide patient follow-up with the addition of tools or online applications for education, processes for written information, and even considerations for billing requirements with telehealth. You may currently see a patient every three months when they make a quarterly visit to the physician's office, but now you have the availability to see them more often. It is vital, however, that the pharmacist continue to have an eye toward the best experience for the patient's needs. While you could provide a full pharmacist appointment every week, that may not be the best use of the patient's time, the pharmacist's time, or finances. However, now is the time to ensure that patients are getting the level of care they need as barriers (i.e., transportation, time off work) are removed. As with face-to-face care, the type of follow-up needed for the patient should be assessed based on the disease state, medication profile, clinical guidelines, and specific patient factors.

- You may find that patients are able to meet the follow-up expectation when the barriers of travel, excess time off work, and so on are removed.
- You may find that your appointment cadence remains the same, but you add touches utilizing remote monitoring, patient portals, or telephone check-ins as you grow your telehealth pharmacy practice offerings.
- You may find that you change the duration of your appointments to larger intervals than before as you have other ways to check in with patients.
- You may find that you change the duration of your appointments to smaller intervals than before for high-risk patients as you have better tools to support appointments outside of the office.

Tools for Telehealth Pharmacy Practice Visit Flow Model: Develop a Streamlined Approach by Planning Steps for Pre-visit, Concurrent/during Visit, and Post-visit Steps

Before the remote visit	• Determine which platform and technology will be used for remote visit. • Ensure the patient has consented to telehealth visit and has necessary technologies. • Determine appropriate space to conduct the visit. • Ensure technology is working. • Confirm patient appointment. • Communicate with clinic staff for a consistent and streamlined care approach.
During the remote visit	• Maintain visual eye contact if completing a tele-video appointment. • Ensure patient readiness and minimize distractions if present. • Conduct the interview and provide clear instructions for any physical assessments needed. • Provide education to patient on assessment and plan using teach-back method.
After the remote visit	• Document in the electronic health record; indicate that visit was performed remotely via telehealth pharmacy practice services. • Provide patient with electronic instructions for follow-up care, medication changes. • Streamline process for access to information post-visit if materials are to be mailed or sent alternatively to electronic follow-up.

SPECIFIC TELEHEALTH PHARMACY PRACTICE EXAMPLES

Heart Failure Telehealth

Heart failure is associated with high morbidity and mortality.[5] Telehealth services in heart failure can reduce hospitalizations and improve overall heart failure symptoms.[6] Successful implementation of these services is contingent on the provider having access to relevant health information and the ability to perform virtual visits for patient assessments. Collection of this information requires utilization of remote technologies that patients can use to transmit data and traditional technologies (e.g., cellphones) to connect patients with providers. Furthermore, heart failure care requires multidisciplinary and interorganizational support. The complexity of care makes clear workflow processes critical to its success. In this section, we outline an example workflow process for heart failure telehealth.

Patient Selection

Remote telehealth for patients with heart failure can be used to triage patients who require urgent care or routine follow-up care.[7] Workflow processes should be developed to triage appropriate care for heart failure patients. For example, patients with Stage D or end-stage heart failure may not be good candidates for virtual visits. These patients may require more physical assessment and multidisciplinary services, given the complex care required. Telehealth can be reserved for patients who require routine heart failure follow-up care (e.g., medication titration, laboratory check, weight and blood pressure assessment). Clear guidance should be provided to identify appropriate patients for telehealth, and whether telehealth is used to help triage patients should be decided.

Clinic Workflow

The heart failure telehealth pharmacy practice visit can flow similarly to a traditional heart failure visit. History taking, medication reconciliation, review of patient vitals, and laboratory measurements can be completed through remote technologies. Ideally, clinical data gathered from remote technologies are prepared in advance for the pharmacist, but they can also be collected during the encounter. Video technology can be used for medication reconciliation and physical examination (e.g., neck veins, peripheral edema, exercise tolerance). At the end of the encounter, the provider–pharmacist team should ensure that the patient receives proper education and communication of the plan. Care should be taken to ensure that referrals are made through proper channels and clearly communicated to the patient. Furthermore, follow-up laboratory and/or diagnostic tests (e.g., echocardiograms, electrocardiograms) need to be coordinated with outside organizations.

Anticoagulation Telehealth Clinic

Telehealth pharmacy practice services for anticoagulation management are well established. A meta-analysis including 15 randomized controlled trials demonstrated that technology-based interventions significantly improved the effectiveness of anticoagulation management.[8] Evaluating time in therapeutic range (TTR), the authors found that patients in the technology-based intervention group had significantly better management compared to that of the control group. Furthermore, major and minor bleeding events were not different between the groups. Home INR testing has been associated with significant improvements in thromboembolic and bleeding events.[9]

Patient Selection

Most patients on anticoagulation can be candidates for remote telehealth pharmacy practice services. Traditionally, these services have been offered to patients on warfarin due to the frequent monitoring warfarin requires, but patients on direct oral anticoagulants can also benefit. Patients on direct oral anticoagulants may benefit from periodic laboratory measurements to check renal function, liver function, adherence monitoring, and safety assessments for signs and symptoms of bleeding.

Clinic Workflow

Workflow for anticoagulation management will depend on the availability of remote monitoring services available to the patient and clinic. Patients on warfarin can obtain INRs from a local laboratory or they can complete home INR testing if available. These data can be gathered prior to the visit to improve workflow efficiency. During the visit, the interview can be conducted to gather remaining patient information. Time should be spent carefully reviewing patient adherence, signs and symptoms of bleeding or thromboembolic complications, and educating the patient on the care plan. Following the encounter, documentation and patient follow-up should be coordinated. The plan should be electronically transmitted to the patient in a secure environment or mailed if that is more appropriate, but with careful consideration regarding what the potential time delay may impose.

Diabetes Telehealth Clinic

Telehealth services in diabetes are also well established. A meta-analysis that included data from 42 randomized controlled trials found that the use of telemedicine led to significant reductions in hemoglobin A1c compared to patients in the usual care group. Older patients (> 50 years) also tended to benefit more when compared to younger patients, dispelling concerns of age-related technological literacy concerns.[10] An abundance of remote monitoring technologies is available to help guide telehealth services in diabetes, including connected glucometers, blood pressure cuffs, and weight scales. These readily available remote monitoring technologies enable the provision of effective telehealth pharmacy practice services.

Patient Selection

The majority of patients living with diabetes are required to perform periodic self-monitoring including blood glucose, blood pressure, weights, and lifestyle assessments. Many remote technologies exist that allow the transfer of data from the patient to the pharmacist. These data can be used to adjust the patient's antihyperglycemic medications to achieve goal HbA1c. Given the wide availability of remote monitoring technologies available, patient selection will be determined primarily by patient willingness to participate and by clinic readiness. Additional consideration may need to be given for new patients versus established patients. Some clinics may prefer in-person visits for new patients since trust as well as confidence for technology literacy need to be developed.

Clinic Work Flow

Collection of data, including self-monitoring blood glucose, blood pressure, and weight, prior to the appointment will improve the efficiency of the telehealth visit. During the visit, patients will need to be instructed on any physical assessment that may be performed (e.g., foot check, retinal exams). Provisions may also need to be made for incorporating specialty providers into the visits. These include dietitians, diabetes educators, or other specialty providers. Careful coordination may be needed if specialty providers are working remotely and not in the same facility.

GROUP TELEHEALTH VISIT TYPES

Some clinics may also decide to incorporate group visits into the telehealth workflow. The use of group visits can improve outcomes by increasing patient engagement and motivation. Group visits typically include 3–20 patients and involve a multidisciplinary team. Group visits are often focused on patient education, shared problem solving, and care coordination.[11] Given the multidisciplinary nature of group visits, coordination of telehealth pharmacy practice services needs to include several different members of the care team (e.g., clinical nurse educator, social worker, physician, medical assistant, and pharmacist). Group visits will require patient consent and utilization of compatible telehealth platforms for all patients involved.

ADDITIONAL SERVICES PROVIDED VIA TELEHEALTH PHARMACY PRACTICE

Medicare Annual Wellness Visits[12]

During the COVID-19 global pandemic, the Centers for Medicare and Medicaid Services (CMS) allowed for Medicare Annual Wellness Visits (AWV) to be adapted to telehealth. While this was likely a temporary measure, it does have benefits for seniors who may not be able to travel to healthcare facilities. It also may allow for providing Medicare AWV services to patients in clinics without access to a pharmacist. As with other appointments, obtaining and documenting vitals or screening tools, as well as providing patient education and written materials, are needed.

For AWV, changes to workflow may be largest within the screening sections. If screening tools are currently completed by support staff in the office, how will they still get completed if the patient and/or the pharmacist is not in the office? In addition, the type of screening tools and your response to the patient's answers may have to be adjusted.

Screening tool examples are as follows:

Cognitive Impairment Assessment:

- If you normally complete a Mini-Cog or other screening tool that requires visual assessment, are you still able to do so via a tele-video visit?
- What assessment tool will you use on a telephone Medicare AWV?
    - The Telephone Intervention for Cognitive Status (TICS) has been recommended for a telehealth visit.

Fall Risk Assessment:

- Is it safe for the patient to complete a physical screening assessment such as a Timed Up and Go (TUG) test while at home without the support of the healthcare team?
    - It has been recommended to consider changing to a question-based fall risk screening for the patient's safety.

Screening for Depression:

- How will you handle a patient screening positive for depression or suicidal risk?
    - How will you handle this if the patient is home with or without additional support?
    - How will you involve your other care team members for support?
        - If during a face-to-face visit you are able to incorporate a physician or a behavioral health team member into the care visit to discuss or provide a quick assessment, how will you provide this service if you are not onsite with those care team members?

Transitions of Care Telehealth Example

The Community Health Network is a large integrated health system in central Indiana serving over 300,000 patients in primary care settings. All pharmacists in the ambulatory care space focus on transitional care management (TCM) for the patients they serve. At the Community Health Network, the goal was always to have a patient complete a postdischarge medication review with a pharmacist as part of value-based care contracts, as well as its known impact on reducing readmission rates.[13] The largest barrier has been coordinating schedules for the pharmacist to see the patient face-to-face prior to the physician or advanced practice provider appointment. The pharmacy team also felt that a telephone review with the loss of assessment for nonverbal cues was not as impactful and noted that the highest risk patients were being prioritized for this pharmacist review.

During the COVID-19 global pandemic, the Community Health Network ambulatory care pharmacy team adjusted to telehealth over the course of 72 hours. With the ability to provide tele-video postdischarge medication reviews, the team felt more confident in transitioning the pharmacist portion of a TCM appointment to a telehealth pharmacy practice encounter. An option remained for a telephone visit if a video visit was not feasible for the patient. During a tele-video visit, the pharmacist was not only able to evaluate a patient's nonverbal cues, but was also able to view pill bottles, assess inhaler and insulin techniques, as well as make other visual assessments that are routine during a face-to-face postdischarge review.

The Community Health Network ambulatory care pharmacy team was able to greatly expand their involvement with postdischarge medication reviews following transitions to tele-video visits. In addition to reaching more of their clinic patients during the postdischarge period, the team expanded to provide postdischarge telehealth pharmacy practice appointments to patients of clinics without a pharmacist and also was able to provide the service to patients following up with a cardiologist in place of or in addition to their primary care provider. In 2019, the team provided 383 postdischarge medication reviews. In 2020, with the addition of a telehealth pharmacy practice focused TCM service, the team completed 1,905 postdischarge medication reviews. This increase represented an almost 400% increase over the previous year.

ADDITIONAL CONSIDERATIONS FOR TELEHEALTH WORKFLOWS

Regardless of whether your workflow for telehealth pharmacy practice appointments looks similar to, or completely different from face-to-face offerings, there are a number of factors to consider when developing your telehealth service. It is important to assess these considerations, as well as any others that may arise in the planning prior to developing the service and at multiple intervals throughout the delivery of the telehealth pharmacy practice service.

Patient-Related Factors

Like any workflow or service, telehealth pharmacy practice services are not one size fits all. As previously mentioned, assessing a patient to ensure telehealth pharmacy practice can meet their needs is an important first step. However, there are additional considerations beyond just deciding if they can receive their pharmacist services via telehealth. Social determinants of health are an important aspect of all of the care provided in an ambulatory care environment. With the addition of telehealth, the gap between patients may widen as those patients with more personal resources may have more access to tools to make telehealth care successful. Here are some considerations for your workflow and planning.

- **Patient resources for telehealth**
    - How will you manage patients without access to a device to allow for video visits?
        - While you may find a need for telephone-based telehealth at times, does telephone alone work for your service?

        - How do you ensure patients receive the same level of care despite their resource differences?
    - If your appointment has a need to screen share, how will this work for patients completing their tele-video visit on their smaller smartphone device?
    - If your patient has a smartphone with limited data, how much data will your tele-video visit consume?
    - If your appointment is sensitive in nature, does the patient have a private space to speak with you?
        - For patients in abusive relationships, how will providing care while they are in their home allow for confidential conversations even if your appointment is not sensitive in nature?
- **Social determinants of health**[14]
    - Economic stability:
        - How does your workflow support all patients regardless of resources at home?
        - How does requesting a patient use their cellphone data plan impact their finances?
    - Healthcare access and quality:
        - How do you provide the same level of service to patients regardless of their resources?
        - If you determine that tele-video visits are the preferred method for your workflow, do you provide an additional hardship to patients without the access to resources?
            - If you determine that patients without access to video visits need to complete face-to-face visits more often, you may be requiring the patients with the least ability to manage transportation barriers to continue to manage those barriers.
        - How can you check a patient's understanding of their healthcare instructions utilizing telehealth?
        - Do you have a process for patients to report poor communication with their pharmacist utilizing telehealth?
        - Do you have access to high-quality interpretive services, and how will you incorporate that in with your telehealth workflow?
    - Social and community context:
        - How is health literacy addressed during telehealth?

Closing Care Gaps in Telehealth

Pharmacists have become integral team members in ambulatory care in part because of their ability to help patients achieve goals. Often, these patient-specific goals are part of a value-based care contract. As billing opportunities continue to lag behind the value pharmacists can provide in ambulatory care, attention to these value-based care contracts measures will be needed to continue to justify the service. Examples of care gaps include a hemoglobin A1c and attention to nephropathy for patients with diabetes, mammograms and colonoscopies for cancer screening, and recommended vaccinations. As patients have less in-person contact with the healthcare team, it is important to develop ways to continue to stress the importance of items that may require face-to-face engagement. Here are some considerations for workflow and planning.

- **Laboratory data**
    - How are you ensuring that labs to help drive the patient care plan and/or needed to close a care gap are still completed?
    - Do you know what labs are important to your value-based care contracts so you can ensure your plans continue to meet these needs?

  - If you are providing point-of-care labs during patient appointments, how will you fill that gap?
    - Could you consider a point-of-care lab day each month where patients can still come to their home physician office for this convenient lab?
      - Could you offer this point-of-care testing in a drive-thru fashion?
    - Could you utilize the support staff still in clinic, for example, a nurse visit for a point-of-care test?
    - Can you partner with lab services to fill this gap?
    - Could you consider the use of at-home point-of-care testing?
    - Do any local retail or independent pharmacies offer point-of-care testing?
  - If the patient cannot travel to a physical site for lab draws, can you collaborate with home health services?
- **Vitals**
  - Do you know what vitals are important to your value-based care contracts to ensure your plans continue to meet these needs?
  - Do you understand what vitals are allowed to be self-reported and how to enter those in your specific EMR?
  - If vitals need to be obtained within the healthcare system, do you have a plan to complete them?
    - Could you consider a "vitals" day each month where patients can still come to their home physician office for this purpose?
      - If so, can you offer this in a drive-thru fashion?
    - Could you utilize the support staff still in clinic, for example, a nurse visit for a vitals check?
    - If the patient cannot travel to a physical site for vitals, can you partner with home health services or utilize remote patient monitoring?
- **Health maintenance**
  - What health maintenance items are important to your value-based care contracts to ensure your plans continue to meet these needs?
  - If face-to-face workflow involves closing health maintenance items, such as during Medicare Annual Wellness Visits, what are the plans to continue to focus on this while utilizing telehealth?
- **Vaccinations**
  - If vaccinations are normally completed during face-to-face visits, what will be the plan for completing vaccinations along with telehealth?
    - Could you consider hosting monthly drive-thru vaccination clinics?
    - Could you partner with a local retail or independent pharmacy?
    - Could you utilize the support staff still in clinic, for example, a nurse visit for a vaccination?

MANAGING CARE TEAM RELATIONSHIPS

Successful ambulatory care pharmacists do not provide care in a silo; rather, they are productive members of a care team. Just as important as the relationship the pharmacist has with their patient, the relationship that the pharmacist has with the rest of the care team is vital to the quality of care they provide. How the pharmacist interacts with the physicians and advanced practice providers in the clinic, as well as nursing and support staff, should be considerations when developing telehealth pharmacy practice workflows.

A benefit to pharmacist-provided telehealth is the ability to expand the reach of pharmacy services. Without telehealth, a pharmacist may be located in one clinic or rotate through a few clinics, but now they could provide a pharmacy service to a much larger patient base. If the current state has a pharmacist rotate between two clinics but the network has eight additional clinics not covered, there are now more tools to expand and provide telehealth pharmacy practice services to the patients of all 10 clinics.

In adjusting a current pharmacy practice experience to include more telehealth services, adjusting the expectations of others in the clinic is another factor to consider. How will providers and staff members be educated regarding the change in delivery method? Another consideration is how will feedback be collected on this offering? If the addition of telehealth pharmacy services leads to covering additional clinic sites or moving the pharmacist offsite, establishing an understanding that pharmacist time will be split between locations can help define expectations. An example of expectations to define may be the availability for helping providers and patients between appointments, as impromptu needs arise for medication education. For example, during face-to-face office encounters, a pharmacist could stop in rooms for new inhaler use education, but if transitioned to remote models, how would these unscheduled needs be managed to maintain optimal care to patients?

If the service is first being offered as a pharmacist telehealth service, establishing care team relationships should be considered essential during the planning discussions, especially if the service is not performed physically onsite with other team members. Planning to meet new team members in person and ensuring involvement with both formal and informal team-building activities could be part of the assessment and planning steps for how to build strong working relationships.

Establishing Expectations

When establishing a telehealth service, there is a need to discuss and clearly outline the patient's expectation for how they are receiving their pharmacist care. Equally vital is establishing expectations with the clinic staff, medical collaborators, and you, individually, as the pharmacist. This first adjustment may be a lot to orient to, but it is important to identify and plan for the fact that it will not be the last adjustment you make to establish an effective and coordinated telehealth pharmacy practice.

When working to adjust patients' expectations for pharmacist care, consider how you define expectations as they pertain to real-time care assessments, flow for appointment, and the overall success of the service for the patient. As patients begin to enjoy the telehealth pharmacy services, how will patient-specific factors be addressed if outlier concerns are raised? Another consideration is how will patients be addressed if they expect all services to be offered remotely if the mixed model is preferred by the clinic?

Regardless of your role on the pharmacy team, there will be a need to look at this new or changing service from a leadership perspective in regard to pharmacy team members providing this remote service. Providing telehealth pharmacy services may not be something that all involved are trained to do. What training will be available to pharmacists and support staff, and how will their ability to work within this new delivery model be assessed? When hiring new staff, will assessments change to address telehealth pharmacy practice skills? A plan for pharmacy learners in this space will also need to be assessed and will be addressed in future chapters.

Clinic workflows need to be redesigned for the provision of telehealth services. In addition to ensuring that the clinic is equipped with telehealth-enabling technology, the clinic must also create workflows that consider staff, provider, and pharmacist responsibilities and physical space. Coordination between organizations must also be considered. Workflow mapping for telehealth services can help identify and anticipate potential barriers and areas where additional support will be needed. Potential barriers for telehealth implementation can be mitigated through clear communication of expectations to both patients and medical staff. With the appropriate resources, telehealth should increase access to care and improve patient satisfaction. Similar to in-person clinic workflows, telehealth pharmacy practice workflows must prioritize patient care and patient safety.

REFERENCES

1. Overview of Workflow Mapping. UCSF Center for Excellence in Primary Care, 2012, **http://cepc.ucsf.edu/sites/cepc.ucsf.edu/files/Overview_workflow_mapping_14-0602.pdf**. Accessed May 16, 2021.
2. Workflow Assessment for Health IT Toolkit. AHRQ. **https://digital.ahrq.gov/health-it-tools-and-resources/evaluation-resources/workflow-assessment-health-it-toolkit/examples**. Accessed May 16, 2021.
3. Practice Facilitation Handbook. Module 5. Mapping and Redesigning Workflow. Content last reviewed May 2013. Agency for Healthcare Research and Quality, Rockville, MD. **http://www.ahrq.gov/professionals/prevention-chronic-care/improve/system/pfhandbook/mod5.html**. Accessed May 16, 2021.
4. National Committee for Quality Assurance. Frequently Asked Questions Directory: HEDIS. **https://www.ncqa.org/hedis/faq/?faq-kw=Blood+pressure&faq-year=&faq-sort=desc&faq-program=**. Accessed May 16, 2021.
5. Orso F, Fabbri G, Maggioni AP. Epidemiology of heart failure. *Handb Exp Pharmacol*. 2017;243:15-33. doi: 10.1007/164_2016_74.
6. Inglis SC, Clark RA, McAlister FA, et al. Which components of heart failure programmes are effective? A systematic review and meta-analysis of the outcomes of structured telephone support or telemonitoring as the primary component of chronic heart failure management in 8323 patients: Abridged Cochrane Review. *Eur J Heart Fail*. 2011 Sep;13(9):1028-1040. doi: 10.1093/eurjhf/hfr039.
7. Gorodeski EZ, Goyal P, Cox ZL, et al. Virtual visits for care of patients with heart failure in the era of COVID-19: A statement from the Heart Failure Society of America. *J Card Fail*. 2020 Jun 1;26(6): 448-456. doi: 10.1016/j.cardfail.2020.04.008.
8. Dai H, Zheng C, Lin C, et al. Technology-based interventions in oral anticoagulation management: Meta-analysis of randomized controlled trials. *J Med Internet Res*. 2020;22(7). **https://www.jmir.org/2020/7/e18386/**
9. Heu M, Welborn T, Nagykaldi Z. In adult patients on warfarin, does home self-testing of prothrombin time and/or international normalized ratio provide the same outcomes compared to testing by a home health nurse or in a clinical setting? *J Okla State Med Assoc*. 2016 Mar;109(3):99-100.
10. Tchero H, Kangambega P, Briatte C, et al. Clinical effectiveness of telemedicine in diabetes mellitus: A meta-analysis of 42 randomized controlled trials. *Telemed E-Health*. 2018 Aug 20;25(7):569-583. doi: 10.1089/tmj.2018.0128.
11. Davis AM, Sawyer DR, Vinci LM. The potential of group visits in diabetes care. *Clin Diabetes*. 2008 Apr 1;26(2):58–62.
12. Hoover M. Adapting the Annual Wellness Visit to Telehealth. **https://caravanhealth.com/CaravanHealth/media/Resources-Page/Telehealth_AWV_AWV-033-20200406-APP.pdf**. Accessed May 16, 2021.
13. Cavanaugh J, Pinell N, Eckel S, et al. Advancing pharmacy practice through an innovative ambulatory care transitions program at an academic medical center. *Pharmacy* 2020;8(1):40. doi: 10.3390/pharmacy8010040.
14. Health People 2030. Social Determinants of Health. **https://health.gov/healthypeople/objectives-and-data/social-determinants-health**. Accessed May 16, 2021.

CHAPTER 5 Description of Operational Telehealth Pharmacy Practice Workflow in Comprehensive Medication Management

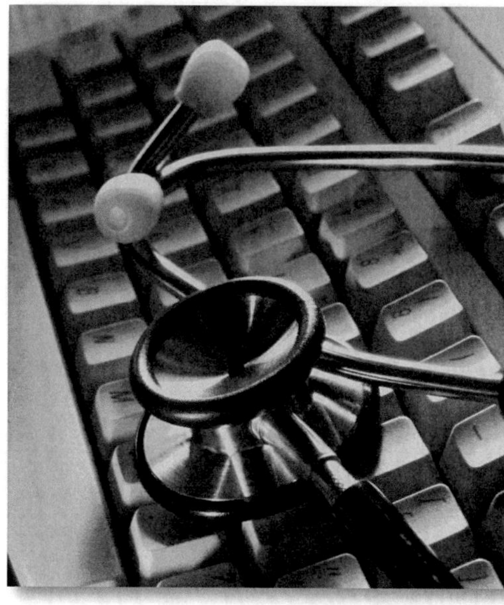

Comprehensive medication management (CMM) is a patient-centered approach to optimizing medication use and improving patient health outcomes that is delivered by a clinical pharmacist working in collaboration with the patient and other healthcare providers. This care process ensures each patient's medications (whether prescription, nonprescription, alternative, traditional, vitamins, or nutritional supplements) are individually assessed to determine that each medication has an appropriate indication, is effective for the medical condition and achieving defined patient and/or clinical goals, and is safe given the comorbidities and other medications being taken. The care process ensures that the patient is able to take the medication as intended and adhere to the prescribed regimen.[1] Three core components of CMM exist for you to consider: a shared philosophy of practice, a patient care process, and a practice management system.[2] These components frame implementation of CMM to your practice regardless of modality.

A shared philosophy of practice serves as a foundation and incorporates the values and beliefs that guide the decisions and actions you will make as part of the interprofessional patient-centered care team.[3] It is critical for you to establish a relationship with both the patient and the provider. This relationship is based on trust and is an essential part of the CMM philosophy. Five core tenets inform the philosophy of practice for CMM. You should embrace these tenets as you integrate CMM into practice.

1. Meeting a social need
2. Assuming responsibility for optimizing medication use
3. Embracing a patient-centered approach
4. Fostering an ongoing patient-pharmacist relationship
5. Working as a collaborative member of the healthcare team

The CMM patient care process occurs when you, working in collaboration with the patient and the healthcare team, provide care to an individual patient with the goal of optimizing medication use and improving the quality of their healthcare.[4] Establishing a common language for the patient care process is essential to ensure that CMM is understood and is valued as distinct from the other care delivered by the team. A standard patient care process also allows the interdisciplinary team of healthcare providers and staff to understand how the ways in which you provide CMM contribute to the patient care process for optimizing medication use. Although the core elements of a patient care process for pharmacists had previously been developed and standards of practice for CMM were published, the

DOI 10.37573/9781585286928.005

CMM in primary care research team sought to apply the principles of implementation science to validate these essential functions of CMM and explicitly describe how to carry out each function.[5] The essential functions of the CMM patient care process include:

1. Collecting and analyzing subjective and objective information
2. Developing and assessing the information to formulate a medication therapy problem list
3. Developing the care plan
4. Implementing the care plan
5. Following up and monitoring, with the goal of ongoing medication optimization and improved care

The operational definitions of each of these essential functions can be found in *The Patient Care Process: A Common Language for Delivering Comprehensive Medication Management*.[4] You are encouraged to review these functions as you provide CMM to ensure fidelity to the true CMM process.

It is important to have a practical assessment of your performance as you deliver CMM. This helps to ensure that the CMM is being implemented as intended.[6] Fidelity to the patient care process when providing CMM is necessary for you to produce optimal patient outcomes; it requires you to take responsibility for optimizing a patient's medications in a manner that is congruent with the work of, and done in collaboration with, the patient's other healthcare providers. Establishing a common language for the provision of CMM has been the key to ensuring that the care provided is consistent and that it is understood by patient, healthcare team, and payers alike.

Finally, you need to consider another component of CMM: the CMM practice management system, which includes regular assessment of the structural and system-level supports needed to effectively implement and sustain a CMM practice.[7] The essential components of practice management are grouped into five domains: organizational support, care delivery processes, care team engagement, evaluation of CMM services, and guarantee of consistent quality care. Organizational support includes having the support of leadership, adequate space for patient care, and financial procedures such as billing. Necessary care delivery processes include methods for identifying those patients needing CMM, patient scheduling, and a system for appropriate documentation. Assessment of care team engagement involves reviewing the presence of a scope of practice or collaborative practice agreement and the extent of interprofessional collaboration, as well as the availability and use of support staff. Evaluation should also include the program's ability to measure and assess data to document that intended outcomes are being achieved. Lastly, guaranteeing consistency and quality of care requires putting quality assurance and improvement processes in place, as well as ongoing CMM practitioner training.

This chapter describes the implementation of CMM using telehealth services. As the philosophy of CMM practice should not change based on the modality of care, we will focus on the intricacies and need for telehealth clinical pharmacy services under the construct of needs related to practice management as well as considerations in the patient care process.

ORGANIZATIONAL SUPPORT

At its foundation, implementing CMM telehealth pharmacy practice starts with organizational support. This includes having the financial means to support the technology platform; having available adequate clinic space for pharmacists to practice; and ensuring services are reimbursed through billing and revenue. Telehealth platforms offer both direct and indirect means for the clinical pharmacist to interact with the patient. A direct relationship includes video, phone, or remote wireless monitoring of a patient. An indirect relationship, however, includes monitoring patients through wearable monitors, mobile apps, and/or web portals.[8] While both relationships offer patients access to 24/7/365 care, the financial means of supporting varies. For some telehealth platforms, the costs of configuration and system setup are included in the institution's license agreement within their EMR. These costs are often associated with a system upgrade. Platforms outside an EMR, however, can be costly for an institution to support and include; there are considerations of security, legality, interface, and quality control. Additionally, having the tech support as well as the personnel to maintain the platform needs to be factored in. While there are many benefits to adopting a platform, the upfront start-up fees can be a deterrent. In contrast, the financial responsibility of indirect relationship telehealth services often falls on the patient, thereby creating a barrier.

Even when direct and indirect telehealth can be financially supported, it is essential that you have adequate space to practice. Fortunately, only minimal space is needed, and typically a clinic room and/or office will suffice. Additionally, adequate light, sound, and privacy are necessary. If one is providing direct patient care through video/phone, a pretest prior to an appointment can be beneficial as part of the steps in pre-visit workflow, as highlighted in Chapter 4. This allows the patient to feel comfortable using the technology prior to the beginning of the appointment. It also helps you as the clinician to troubleshoot any connection or environmental barriers the patient may be experiencing. One of the few studies available—Hatton et al.—studied the correlation between direct telehealth services and patient satisfaction.[9] Through a 30- to 45-minute face-to-face video-conference, patients interacted with a pharmacist to review their medication therapies. Post-interaction, patients were asked to complete a Likert Scale questionnaire. Results showed a positive correlation between telehealth pharmacy practice services and patient satisfaction. Once patients felt comfortable using the video device, patient-centered communication scored just as high as or higher than direct face-to-face visits.

Even if patient satisfaction is positive and an institution can provide financial support, billing and revenue associated with services is key. Payers have proposed different models for payment, including fee-for-service as well as capitated. Some payers differentiate between services such as telehealth phone versus video-conferencing. However, as the marketplace continues to shift and the need for minimal exposure increases, some payers may begin to favor or even mandate such service. This development would certainly shift the reimbursement on many levels. (Refer to Section 3, Exploring Revenue Opportunities with Telehealth for Pharmacists.)

CARE DELIVERY PROCESS FOR CMM

Developing the care delivery process of CMM telehealth pharmacy practice services involves many considerations and stakeholders. Once a service is selected, a team involving implementation experts, IT support, and end users needs to be created. Often, super users are identified who aid in testing and training colleagues once live. At University of Wisconsin (UW) Health, virtual telehealth appointments were quickly launched to support COVID-driven needs. Super users—providers in specialty ambulatory clinics—were identified and taken offline for several days to train and be the first to support their patient panels on telehealth video-conferencing. Within the Carbone Cancer Center, caregivers, including pharmacists who worked directly with providers involved with telehealth, were also trained. During implementation, workflows were created to determine which oncology patients were eligible for telehealth and how each visit would be scheduled. Patients considered for telehealth oncology services included those who (1) had established care with the provider; (2) were not initiating therapy; and (3) were active in their electronic medical record. Prior to go-live, "test runs" were performed with mock patients to ensure that connectivity and interfacing worked properly. The marketing team at UW Health also created end-user guides and videos for patients to reference prior to their appointments. These guides were automatically sent through email and/or EMR once a video conference had been scheduled. Those who were not active on their EMR had more difficulty connecting with telehealth services. This clear barrier was highlighted during this process.

Prior to a patient tele-video conference beginning, a medical assistant logged into the remote video room to test connectivity with the patient. Providers, nurses, and pharmacists were then able to join in/out of the remote room during the visit. In total, patient visits were 30–40 minutes in length. Afterward, patients would log out of the remote room, and providers would document the encounter in the patient's EMR. The encounter was then signed, closed, and billed to the payer as a telehealth visit. Since pharmacists cannot bill for services directly in Wisconsin, their time spent with the patient was accounted for in the overall visit.

To date, CMM telehealth pharmacy practice services continue to increase. Within the next five years, some institutions are projecting that telehealth services will account for 30–50% of ambulatory clinic encounters. While this projection may seem encouraging, many barriers remain and need to be considered. For one, a quality control plan for how to operate during downtime needs to be created and tested. In the event of a network or EMR outage, institutions must know if video-conferencing would still be available "offline." Additionally, from a security standpoint, third-party platforms need to be continually monitored for quality assurance to verify patient information remains confidential. Despite challenges, telehealth will remain a viable care modality for the future. Influenced by key market trends, telehealth aligns with (1) continuing innovation in a consumer-driven technology market, (2) supporting advancement in EMR and clinical decision support, and (3) improving care delivery and access.[8]

MULTIDISCIPLINARY CARE TEAM MANAGEMENT FOR CMM

As mentioned above, the entire care team is involved in CMM telehealth pharmacy practice services. While this will be expanded upon in the next section, interprofessional collaboration and appropriate training are necessary to support such services. Sharma et al.[10] suggest the need for provider training in a virtual communication and website manner. Mannerisms such as hand gestures or body positioning can distract a patient from their appointment. Additionally, communicating too quickly may cause more confusion and be difficult to follow in a remote platform. Suggestions to incorporate CMM telehealth training during medical school and residency are now widely endorsed.[10] This training is essential not only for providers, but for pharmacists, nurses, and medical assistants as well.

EVALUATION AND QUALITY IMPROVEMENT PROCESSES

CMM Provided by Telehealth

The evaluation of CMM services via telehealth pharmacy practice offers many similarities compared to the evaluation of any CMM service.[7] Evaluation of CMM provided by telehealth allows you to focus on continual improvement and refinement of the overall program. As discussed earlier, CMM evaluation can be broken down into activities that assess the program management components to include organizational support, care delivery processes, care team engagement, evaluating CMM services, and ensuring consistent quality care. This evaluation will span different stages to include the implementation and sustainment phases ranging from pre-implementation, implementation to stabilization, and following a normal plan, do, study, and act (PDSA) process.[6]

Traditionally, much focus has been placed on the evaluation of CMM telehealth services related to the achievement of only specific clinical biomarkers with pharmacist care. There are more components of evaluation of a CMM telehealth practice other than clinical biomarkers alone that include different perspectives to include the patient, the provider, and the payer.

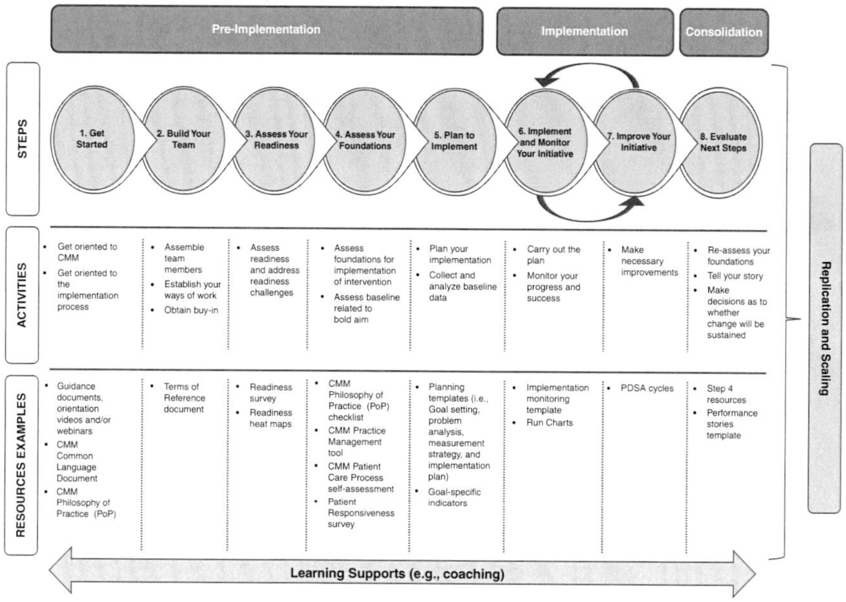

Source: Used with permission from the CMM in Primary Care Research Team.

Evaluation of the Practice Management Components of CMM Telehealth

The practice management components of CMM are those components that support the ability for you to provide CMM in an effective, efficient, and productive manner. In a study intended to identify the core components of CMM practices, the CMM primary care study team evaluated 35 mature CMM practices with embedded clinical pharmacists across the country.[6] As part of the completion of this work, the team created a practice management assessment tool (PMAT), which allows assessment and prioritization for improvement in the practice management areas of CMM. The assessment includes the core practice management components related to CMM and sets the standard for evaluation of the practice management components related to CMM regardless of modality. Additionally, in 2018, the team released the *Patient Care Process for Delivering CMM*. This publication, modeled on the Joint Commission on Pharmacy Practice Patient Care Process, was developed after looking at common themes in the 35 practices.[5] The practice management components of CMM for telehealth must be evaluated at some level as they set the foundation for the pharmacist to achieve positive results in any of the other outcomes measured.

Evaluation of Process Measures of CMM Telehealth

Process measures are those metrics that evaluate what any provider does to maintain or improve health.[11] For you and CMM telehealth services, collecting baseline process data is required in order to maintain a longitudinal, prospective evaluation. Given that CMM telehealth pharmacy practice services have the ability to increase access to care, process measures evaluating access should be at the forefront. In a study conducted by the Department of Veterans Affairs, clinical pharmacist services provided by clinical video telehealth (CVT) were compared to face-to-face services provided in a single outpatient clinic.[12] The study evaluated the potential benefits of telehealth pharmacy practice to include an increase in access, which took in the time from request of visit to appointment, and average travel distance and average travel time averted. The average time in days from consult placement to initial visit decreased from 106.3 ± 24.5 to 46 ± 35.3 (p <0.0001). The average travel distance in miles averted per patient was 99.5 ± 20.3, and the average travel time in hours averted was 1.6 ± 0.3. In addition, no-show rates with telehealth services were 4% as compared to 10% with face-to-face care.[12]

Suggested access process metrics for CMM telehealth pharmacy practice services are as follows:

- Time to completion of an appointment from requested date (i.e., new patient and established patient wait times)
- No-show rates
- Clinic utilization of telehealth CMM appointments
- Number of visits per individual patient
- Supply versus demand for CMM telehealth appointments

Evaluation of the above access process measures allow pharmacy leadership to evaluate and proactively improve and/or anticipate opportunities. For example, if new patient wait times for a CMM telehealth pharmacy practice appointment are extended, evaluation of the supply of appointments and no-show rates could be considered in order to target and possibly generate additional care opportunities or project the need for additional telehealth appointments. Evaluation of access processes may reveal foundational programmatic practice management deficiencies. For example, if clinic utilization of telehealth appointments is low while no-show rates for appointments are high, it could uncover issues related to appointment scheduling and/or appointment reminders for patients (i.e., pre-visit appointment workflow). Process measures for access and foundational components of practice management are directly proportional. Strategies could then be implemented to decrease no-show rates to increase clinic utilization and subsequently access availability.

Additional process measures for CMM telehealth pharmacy practice services include pharmacist productivity related to CMM. Your productivity can include total time spent in patient care, number of patient care encounters in relation to time spent in patient care, number of medication therapy problems (MTP) identified, and the interventions provided during the patient care encounter. Pharmacist productivity should be individualized to the direct patient time of the pharmacist, which may include preparatory activities. Evaluation of interventions can include specific activities related to disease states, types and acceptance for interventions, and ordering activities, including laboratories, medication, or referrals. For example, if a need of care is identified for substance use disorder and an evaluation of practice reveals most telehealth services provided are focused on diabetes, a reeducation or pivot in care focus to more comprehensive management should be pursed. Individual healthcare system or facility evaluation will differ based on the resources available to evaluate. However, processes to evaluate productivity of pharmacists providing telehealth should be integrated into evaluation of CMM processes. Lastly, modality of telehealth care in regard to pharmacist productivity may also be considered. Some pharmacists may participate more in traditional telephonic care, while other pharmacists may provide telehealth pharmacy practice through a video modality. Given the complexities of video technology (e.g., bandwidth) efficiency, providing a telehealth visit may vary. Individual healthcare systems or practices must decide and individualize productivity based on these considerations.

Fiscal components of a telehealth CMM program must be evaluated and include such measures as generated revenue and/or cost savings from a CMM program. A thorough discussion of fiscal measures is provided in Section 3.

EVALUATION OF CLINICAL OUTCOMES OF CMM TELEHEALTH

Creation of strategies related to the clinical outcomes of care and its monitoring are highly recommended. Evaluation of clinical outcomes allows for quantification if the process for patient care delivery has already achieved, or is achieving, the intended outcome for patient care. Evaluation of clinical care goes far beyond developing randomized controlled trials or retrospective analysis for publication. Evaluation of clinical outcomes answers the question, "Is the patient receiving the benefit intended from the services I am providing?"

Developing clinical outcomes for CMM should be individualized and if possible be specific to the care you are providing. Outcomes should be comprehensive, scientifically sound, and usable for improvement. Many clinical outcomes may be either completely or partially influenced by you or must be surrogate metrics for care. For example, in a true team-based model, you will not be the only person contributing to the care of the patient, which at times may provide heterogeneity to evaluation of a quality metric. Regardless, whenever possible, it is important to provide granularity to the care you are providing when possible. Several organizations have created metrics that, while not specific to CMM and telehealth, can be utilized to evaluate CMM.[13-19]

Multiple meta-analysis and systematic reviews have highlighted the benefits of pharmacy provider care.[20,21] Specific to telehealth pharmacy practice, a telehealth-based chronic disease management program evaluated the impact on specific primary care outcomes.[22] Patients were targeted for diabetes, hypertension, and tobacco cessation. Patients in the diabetes and hypertension groups had a mean absolute HbA1c reduction of 1.61% (95% confidence interval [CI], 1.39–1.83%; p <0.0001) and a mean systolic blood pressure reduction of 26.00 mm Hg (95% CI, 22.99-28.50 mm Hg; p <0.001), respectively. Tobacco cessation was achieved in 42% of targeted patients. Similarly, blood pressure control was evaluated in 156 patients in a home-based-digital-medicine blood pressure program compared to 400 patients in a usual care group. Mean decrease in systolic/diastolic blood pressure was 14/5 mm Hg in digital medicine versus 4/2 mm Hg in usual care (p <0.001).[23]

Although a comprehensive list of quality metrics for telehealth and CMM does not currently exist, utilization of currently published metrics for evaluation of quality of care can be extrapolated to CMM in telehealth. A complete list of metrics evaluated should be individualized at the healthcare system level, but these can include but not be limited to measures that report adherence to medications, appropriate use of medications, medication safety, and overall clinical measures. Examples of metrics that could be considered include but are not limited to:

- Medication possession ratios for specific classes of medications
- Statin use in patients with diabetes or cardiovascular disease
- Percent of patients on high-dose opioids
- Blood pressure control <140/90 mmHg
- HbA1c testing done annually
- Diabetes control with HbA1c <8%
- Disease state specific 30-day readmission rates postdischarge
- Beta blocker use post-myocardial infarct
- ACE-I/ARB use in heart failure

EVALUATION OF PATIENT EXPERIENCE AND PROVIDER SATISFACTION OF CMM TELEHEALTH

Evaluation of patient experience with CMM is a relatively new offering. The Consumer Assessment of Healthcare Providers and Systems (CAHPS) has been used as the measure to evaluate a patient's experience, both inpatient and outpatient, related to access, provider responsiveness and satisfaction, and overall patient satisfaction. A study specific to evaluation of satisfaction using CAHPS for pediatric patients seen by an advanced practice nurse showed that telehealth improved overall ratings of caregiver experience with healthcare providers.[24] Although these data are useful for an overall viewpoint related to patient satisfaction, this information is not specific to a clinical pharmacist providing CMM. A study published in 2015 evaluated the impact of a pharmacist-led telehealth clinic on diabetes-related goals of therapy.[12] As part of this study, the investigators evaluated the level of patient satisfaction with pharmacist care and with the telehealth modality using a modified version of the Satisfaction with Pharmacists (SWiP) scale. Patient satisfaction scores were very high overall, with a median score of 39.5 (Interquartile range [IQR] 36–40) out of a maximum score of 40. In addition, Barr and colleagues revealed higher patient engagement in hypertension management with a clinical pharmacist and a health coach using a home-based blood pressure program.[25]

Continued research related to patient satisfaction and CMM specific with telehealth is needed. However, evaluation of patient satisfaction is a must in relation not only to access of care but also to the modality of care provider.

Provider satisfaction with CMM services, specifically telehealth, is lacking. However, studies regarding CMM integration have shown positive effects on provider well-being by decreasing workload.[26] Funk and colleagues conducted a series of structured interviews with 16 primary care providers where CMM was implemented. Providers reported a decrease in mental exhaustion resulting from the reassurance of having a clinical pharmacy colleague to consult and to provide enhanced opportunities for professional learning. McFarland and colleagues evaluated provider perceptions after integrating a clinical pharmacist providing CMM into practice. Using a Likert Scale of 1 being poor perception and 5 being significant contribution on evaluation of whether integration of pharmacists into the PACT model "improve(s) your job satisfaction," the overall rating was 4.29 with nurse practitioners, physicians, and nurses rating pharmacists at 4.67, 4.59, and 4.43, respectively.[26] Provider satisfaction with CMM telehealth services should be highly considered as part of a CMM telehealth evaluation.

REPORTING CMM TELEHEALTH DATA

Extracting CMM data in an efficient and reproducible manner is crucial. As outlined above, metrics can be classified as clinical, access, patient, and provider satisfaction. Extracting data will vary depending on the healthcare system or individual practice. Regardless of practice, it is highly recommended, when possible, that data be accumulated in a proficient and reproducible manner. The use of manual chart extraction for clinical metrics, when possible, should be streamlined, with the hopes that electronic processes can be in place through automated reports for you to use. The data generated should be evaluated for the CMM program as a whole, but they should be able to be evaluated down to the patient level.

Once outcome data have been chosen and evaluated, use of the data is crucial to ensure that improvements and/or demonstration of benefit are provided. You and the team should have plans in place to evaluate the overall outcomes garnered and either used to demonstrate the value of CMM and telehealth or areas of improvement. These data, once gathered, can be presented internally to the team where the patient is seeking care, facility, or healthcare leadership, or you may present externally to payers and/or at professional meetings/publication. Pharmacy leaders should have scheduled times (i.e., quarterly, monthly) when this information is reported.

Ensuring Consistent Quality Care

Establishing evaluation components to ensure quality of care for telehealth CMM is important. Basic activities that you provide related to CMM via telehealth (e.g., the patient care process) should not differ from face-to-face care. However, training processes should be in place to ensure that new staff or current staff entering into the telehealth arena or exploring new technology should be in place. This could include a mentoring program where a high-functioning pharmacist with telehealth mentors a new or struggling pharmacist. In addition, ongoing developments related to telehealth could be considered during staff meetings, journal clubs, or other group settings. Facility or healthcare system policies should be routinely updated to address changes in facility, state, and/or federal regulations related to telehealth management. These changes should be routinely relayed to the provider practicing CMM in the telehealth environment. Lastly, data generated from CMM telehealth outcomes should be incorporated into a quality assessment process. This could include pharmacy-specific activities or activities addressed by a facility quality assurance team.

REFERENCES

1. Patient-Centered Primary Care Collaborative (PCPCC). The patient-centered medical home: Integrating comprehensive medication management to optimize patient outcomes resource guide, 2nd ed. Washington, DC: PCPCC, 2012. **www.pcpcc.org/sites/default/files/media/medmanagement.pdf**. Accessed May 16, 2021.
2. Livet M, Blanchard C, Frail C, et al. Ensuring effective implementation: A fidelity assessment system for comprehensive medication management. *J Am Coll Clin Pharm.* 2020;3:57-67. **https://doi.org/10.1002/jac5.1155**.
3. Pestka DL, Sorge LA, McClurg MR, Sorensen TD. The philosophy of practice for comprehensive medication management: Evaluating its meaning and application by practitioners. *Pharmacotherapy.* 2018;38(1):69-79. **https://doi.org/10.1002/phar.2062**.
4. Joint Commission of Pharmacy Practitioners. Pharmacists' Patient Care Process. May 29, 2014. **https://jcpp.net/wp-content/uploads/2016/03/PatientCareProcess-with-supporting-organizations.pdf**. Accessed May 16, 2021.
5. The Patient Care Process for Delivering Comprehensive Medication Management (CMM): Optimizing Medication Use in Patient-Centered, Team-Based Care Settings. CMM in Primary Care Research Team. July 2018. **http://www.accp.com/cmm_care_process**. Accessed May 16, 2021.
6. Livet M, Blanchard C, Sorenson TD, McClurg MR. An implementation system for medication optimization: Operationalizing comprehensive medication management delivery in primary care. *J Am Coll Clin Pharm.* 2018;1(1):14-20. **https://doi.org/10.1002/jac5.1037**.
7. Pestka DL, Frail CK, Sorge LA, et al. Development of the comprehensive medication management practice management assessment tool: A resource to assess and prioritize areas for practice improvement. *J Am Coll Clin Pharm.* 2019;3(2):448-454. **https://doi.org/10.1002/jac5.1182**.
8. Tuckson RV, Edmunds M, Hodgkins ML. Telehealth. *N Engl J Med.* 2017;377(16):1585-1592. doi: 10.1056/NEJMsr1503323.
9. Hatton J, Chandra R, Lucius D, et al. Patient satisfaction of pharmacist-provided care via clinical video teleconferencing. *J Pharm Pract.* 2018;31(5):429-433. doi: 10.1177/0897190017715561.
10. Sharma R, Nachum S, Davidson KW, Nochomovitz M. It's not just FaceTime: Core competencies for the medical virtualist. *Int J Emerg Med.* 2019;12(1):8. Published 2019 Mar 12. doi:10.1186/s12245-019-0226-y.
11. AHRQ. Improving survey response rates to get actionable data. **https://beterra.com/solutions/safeculture/ahrq-hsops-mosops/**. Accessed May 16, 2021.
12. Maxwell LG, McFarland MS, Baker JW, Cassidy RF. Evaluation of the impact of a pharmacist-led telehealth clinic on diabetes-related goals of therapy in a veteran population. *Pharmacotherapy.* 2016;36(3):348-356. **https://doi.org/10.1002/phar.1719**.
13. Pharmacy Quality Alliance. Strategies to expand value-based pharmacist-provided care action guide for community pharmacists, healthcare payers, and other stakeholders. **https://pqa.memberclicks.net/assets/S2S/Pharmacist-Provided%20Care%20Action%20Guide.pdf**. Accessed May 16, 2021.
14. Pharmacy Quality Alliance. Access to care: Development of a medication access framework for quality measurement. **https://www.pqaalliance.org/assets/Research/PQA-Access-to-Care-Report.pdf**. March 2019. Accessed May 16, 2021.
15. Pharmacy Quality Alliance. PQA measure use in CMS' part D quality programs. **https://www.pqaalliance.org/medicare-part-d**. Accessed May 16, 2021.
16. National Committee for Quality Assurance. HEDIS and Performance Measures. **https://www.ncqa.org/hedis/**. Accessed May 16, 2021.
17. Andrawis M, Ellison C, Riddle S, et al. Recommended quality measures for health-system pharmacy: 2019 update from the Pharmacy Accountability Measures Work Group. *Am J Health Syst Pharm.* 2019;76:874-888. doi: 10.1093/ajhp/zxz069.
18. Agency for Healthcare Research and Quality. CAHPS: Assessing healthcare quality from the patient's perspective. **https://www.ahrq.gov/sites/default/files/wysiwyg/cahps/about-cahps/cahps-program-brief.pdf**. Accessed May 16, 2021.
19. Clements, JN, Emmons, RP, Anderson, SL, et al. Current and future state of quality metrics and performance indicators in comprehensive medication management for ambulatory care pharmacy practice. *J Am Coll Clin Pharm.* 2021;4:390-405. **https://doi.org/10.1002/jac5.1406**.

20. Tan ECK, Stewart K, Elliott RA, George J. Pharmacist services provided in general practice clinics: A systematic review and meta-analysis. *Res Social Adm Pharm* 2014;10(4):608-622. doi: 10.1016/j.sapharm.2013.08.006.
21. Greer N, Bolduc J, Geurkink E, et al. Pharmacist-led chronic disease management: A systematic review of effectiveness and harms compared to usual care. *Ann Intern Med.* 2016;165(1):30-40. doi: 10.7326/M15-3058.
22. Litke J, Spoutz L, Ahlstrom D, et al. Impact of the clinical pharmacy specialist in telehealth primary care. *Am J Health Syst Pharm.* 2018 Jul 1;75(13):982-986. doi: 10.2146/ajhp170633.
23. Bangalore S, Toklu B, Gianos E, et al. Optimal systolic blood pressure target after SPRINT: Insights from a network meta-analysis of randomized trials. *Am J Med.* 2017 Jan;130(1):14-20. doi: 10.1016/j.amjmed.2016.07.029.
24. Looman W, Antolick M, Cady R. Effects of a telehealth care coordination intervention on perceptions of health care by caregivers of children with medical complexity: A randomized controlled trial. *J Pediatr Health Care.* Jul-Aug 2015;29(4):352-363. doi:.10.1016/j.pedhc.2015.01.007.
25. Barr PJ, Forcino RC, Thompson R, et al. Evaluating collaborate in clinical setting: Analysis of mode effects on scores, response rates and costs of data collection. *J Med Internet Res.* 2014 Jan 3;16(1):e2. doi: 10.2196/jmir.3085.
26. McFarland MS, Lamb K, Hughes J, et al. Perceptions of integration of the clinical pharmacist into the patient care medical home model. *J Healthcare Quality.* 2018;40(5):265-273. **https://doi.org/10.1097/jhq.0000000000000114**.

SECTION 2: CLINICAL VIGNETTE

Scenario 1

You recently started a position as clinical pharmacist at a physician-based clinic located in a rural area. Since starting, you have implemented chronic disease management services for diabetes, hypertension, and dyslipidemia. To date, you have a no-show rate of approximately 45%, and many patients state it is simply too far to travel from their home for monthly appointments. Given this significant no-show rate and identified barrier, you would like to explore establishing telehealth pharmacy services. Who could you reach out to as a first step to discuss this opportunity?

Response 1

The clinic manager would be a great resource for you when considering starting telehealth pharmacy services. The clinic manager will likely know about any current telehealth services and workflows that could be extended to include telehealth pharmacy services. If there are no existing telehealth services or workflows, the clinic manager would be a necessary partner for helping to establish telehealth pharmacy services. For example, the clinic manager will be able to engage key staff members in needed workflows such as patient check-in or registration, enrolling patients in the telehealth platform or providing support or education on a telehealth platform, scheduling, and so on. It can also be beneficial to have a physician champion involved in the process to help advocate for the importance of pharmacy services to have access and resources to provide telehealth pharmacy services.

Scenario 2

While working through developing workflows for telehealth pharmacy services, you become concerned about the ability to have your patient share any blood sugar or home blood pressure monitoring data in a meaningful way. You are concerned about having to work through a month's worth of data with patients either over the phone or virtually to get the information you need to make adjustments to medication regimens. Plus, you are worried that getting all that information during the visit may take up a significant portion of the visit time.

Response 2

Review what options you could build into your workflow to capture patient-reported data prior to the telehealth visit. Some electronic health records may capture patient-reported data. This could occur through asynchronous modalities such as patient messaging or flow-sheets that have prespecified fields for patient responses. If there are no options to leverage within the electronic health record to obtain these data pre-visit, consider what other options may be available: for example, leveraging clinical staff to call patients ahead of their telehealth pharmacy appointment to gather pertinent information, including the data needed for clinical decision making during the visit.

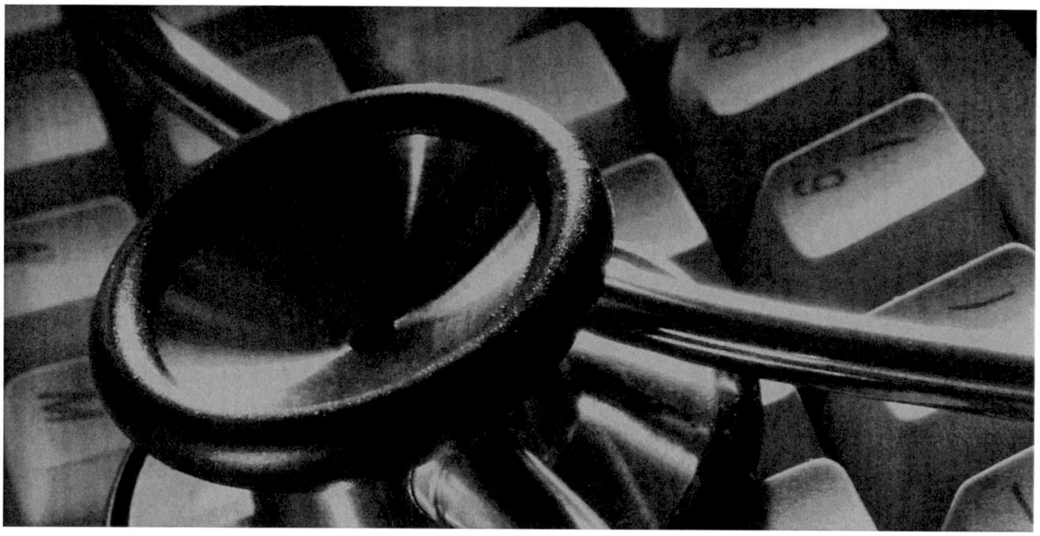

SECTION 3
Exploring Revenue Opportunities with Telehealth for Pharmacists

Mary Ann Kliethermes, Jennifer Reiter, and Brody Maack

CHAPTER 6 Foundational Elements of Billing for Telehealth Pharmacy Practice

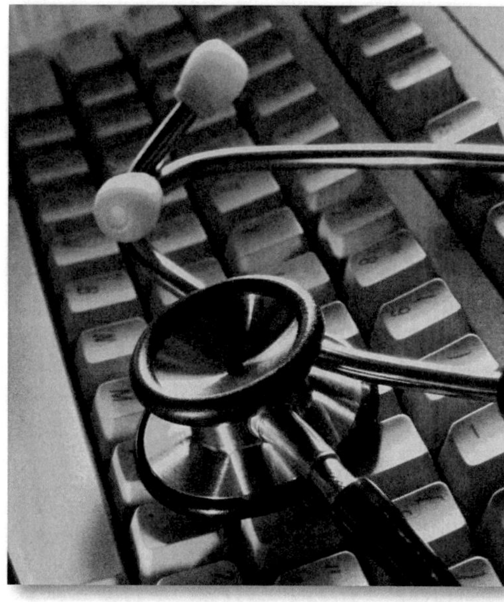

UNDERSTANDING BILLING BASICS

Obtaining reimbursement for pharmacist patient care services directly or indirectly is a challenging endeavor. In the fee-for-service model, which remains prevalent as the major healthcare payment structure, obtaining sufficient renumeration for pharmacist patient care services requires a patchwork of allowable billing options. Unfortunately, many of the billing choices do not match well to the breadth and depth of services provided by many pharmacists. Adding telehealth to the reimbursement patchwork further magnifies the complexity.

Today's healthcare environment requires providers, including pharmacists, not only to pay attention to their costs and revenue generation to sustain their practices, but also to demonstrate the value of their services by its contribution to their patients' health outcomes. Consequently, pharmacists, regardless of their practice settings, should have a solid understanding of the basics of medical billing and healthcare revenue generation. Doing so enables you to navigate the communication bridge with billers, administrators, compliance officers, and payer personnel as you embark to secure reimbursement and overcome the numerous barriers to maximize the revenue-generating capabilities of your service.

Direct reimbursement to pharmacists for patient care services remains uncommon, existing in only a handful of states across the country and for a few billing codes at the federal level. For direct reimbursement to occur, benefit policies need to recognize pharmacists as legal healthcare providers, and benefit plans need to cover pharmacist services. Although many states and the District of Columbia have statutes that classify pharmacists as healthcare providers,[1] the ability to bill for services remains unavailable in most states. Reimbursement hinges on three criteria governed by legislative action at the state level.[2]

1. Pharmacists by legislation and rule are recognized as healthcare providers in the state.
2. The services pharmacists provide and bill are clearly described under a defined scope of practice within the state pharmacy practice act.
3. Insurance laws direct commercial health plans to include pharmacists as a provider eligible to bill and receive payment for patient care services within the payer's benefit plans and within the pharmacist's scope of practice.

Without each of these criteria in place, pharmacists must rely on generating revenue by partnering with authorized billing providers who are able to delegate and then bill for services delivered by a pharmacist designated as ancillary services to the care they provide.

DOI 10.37573/9781585286928.006

Healthcare Payers

The initial step in determining how to generate revenue for your services is to determine your payer mix or the major healthcare payers for your patient population. Reimbursement amounts and rules will differ among payers, and you will want to maximize your revenue options from those payers that insure most of your patient population. In the United States, healthcare services are primarily paid for by government at the federal and state level and commercial payers. For the typical ambulatory care provider, commercial payers compose the largest payer group at 43%, with Medicare the second largest at 29% and state Medicaid at 17%.[3] Contributing to a lesser degree are self-pay patients, or smaller payers such as workers' compensation. Geographic location of your practice will greatly influence your payer mix, for urban, suburban, and rural practices will differ in the age and economic makeup and thus the insurer of the population. For most practices, Medicare is the largest single payer and one reason most payment strategies focus on Medicare.

Tool for telehealth pharmacy practice billing: Reach out to billing staff and/or financial administrators in your health system or at your local clinic(s). Most will be willing to share the specific payer mix of their patient population to help guide you in identifying billable services.

Commercial Payers

The commercial payer group is composed of many entities offering a myriad of benefit plans that can differ greatly in services covered. State laws and rules mandate what commercial payers licensed in their state are required to provide as benefits to all beneficiaries, to which providers must be paid for providing those services within the providers' state scope of practice. State laws and rules mandate what commercial payers licensed in their state are required to provide as minimal healthcare benefits to all state residents, which providers must be paid for providing those services if they are within their state scope of practice. With the variety and variability in commercial plans, it is difficult to provide specific guidance on the best strategy to secure payment for pharmacist services. You may wish to work with your organization to identify the commercial health plans that predominate in your population and propose developing specific contracts with the payers to cover your services with agreed-upon service billing codes. Though not widespread, these types of payment models do exist in the commercial space. When no specific contract exists, commercial payers follow the rules of the industry standard billing system, which is the Medicare billing system.

Tool for telehealth pharmacy practice billing: If you find many of your patients are employed by a specific company, it can be helpful to reach out to the employer to discuss services you can provide. The employer can work with you and their insurance provider to develop a method for providing reimbursable services.

State Medicaid

Medicaid is a state-run program that provides healthcare coverage for people with extremely low or no income. Medicaid is jointly funded by the state and federal government, where the federal government matches state funding based on a specified percentage of program expenditures, called the federal medical assistance percentage (FMAP). FMAPs range from 50 to 75%, with an average of 57%, and are adjusted every three years. For states that expand Medicaid under the Affordable Care Act, the federal government assumes 100% of the FMAP for a set number of years for the added beneficiaries. Individual states construct their own Medicaid benefit plans and provider reimbursement rates within federal requirements and use either a fee-for-service or a managed care model in administering benefits. Thus, there is variability in rules and regulations regarding pharmacists' ability to bill and be reimbursed. Fourteen state Medicaid programs offer some level of direct reimbursement to pharmacists for patient care services, and reimbursement for telehealth pharmacy practice services varies among these states (**Table 6.1**).[4] All 14 states are authorized for Medicaid reimbursement of live video telehealth, but only three states (Minnesota, Missouri, and Oregon) allow reimbursement for three forms of telehealth (live video, store-and-forward, and remote

Table 6.1. States with Medicaid Reimbursement for Pharmacist Patient Care Services, and Corresponding Telehealth Medicaid Reimbursement

	Medicaid Reimbursement for Telehealth		
States	Live Video	Store-and-Forward	Remote Patient Monitoring
California	√	√	
Colorado	√		√
Georgia	√	√	
Iowa	√		
Kansas	√		√
Michigan	√		
Minnesota	√	√	√
Missouri	√	√	√
New Mexico	√	√	
North Dakota	√		
Ohio	√		
Oregon	√	√	√
Washington	√	√	
Wisconsin	√		

patient monitoring).[5] If Medicaid is a major payer for your population, consult the state regulations where you practice for the rules on billing and reimbursement for pharmacist patient care services.

A specific group of Medicaid beneficiaries, termed "dual eligible," is eligible for Medicare benefits but is also of extremely low income and qualify for Medicaid as a secondary payer that assumes payment for any Medicare copay the beneficiary accrues. Dual-eligible patients are considered a high-risk population for both medical conditions and cost.

Medicare

Medicare is the federal government's health insurance program available to any U.S. citizen or legal resident (or their spouse) who has paid at least 10 years of taxes into Medicare through their employment and has been a citizen or legal resident in the United States for a minimum of 5 years. Health coverage begins when a person reaches 65 years of age or older or has become medically disabled. Medicare benefits are established through legislative action by the U.S. Congress, which began with the Social Security Act in 1965 and many subsequent laws since. By law, Medicare Part A and Part B plans cover 80% of any billable service and require the patient to be responsible for the remaining 20%. Patients may have coinsurance that assists in covering the 20% co-pay. This may be in the form of private retirement health insurance benefits, Medigap plans, or state Medicaid coverage in the dual-eligible population.

Table 6.2 summarizes four Medicare benefit plans. The Center for Medicare and Medicaid Services (CMS) is the federal agency under Health and Human Services whose role is to administer

Table 6.2. Medicare Benefits Summary

Benefit Design	Medicare A	Medicare B	Medicare C	Medicare D
Type	Universal	Opt-out	Opt-in	Opt-out
Coverage	Hospital care Long-term care Some home health	Outpatient services Durable medical equipment Preventive services Ambulance services Some home health	Must include Part A and Part B May add other services • Prescription • Eye care • Dental • Hearing • Other	Prescription Medications
Annual Rules Document(s)	IPPS (Inpatient Prospective Payment System)	PFS (physician fee schedule) HOPPS (Hospital Outpatient Prospective Payment System)	CMS Call Letter	CMS Call Letter MTM Program Guidance Memo
Timing of call for annual comments to the final rule	April–October	July–November	January–May	January–May
CMS Payment	*To Hospitals based on:* *MS-DRGs (Medical Severity Diagnosis-Related Groups)* *Revenue codes* *Quality Metrics*	To eligible providers for services and procedures using HCPC codes Quality Metrics	To contracted commercial payer Quality Metrics	To contracted PDP Quality Metrics

Medicare benefits and set the rules and regulations for how each plan is administered. It is important to be aware of who CMS pays under each plan and the documents that annually update the rules and regulations for each benefit. Knowing who gets paid directs you to the organization or providers pharmacists must speak with to secure reimbursement for services provided to the Medicare's plan patient population. The rule document will provide what is allowable by CMS for generating revenue as pharmacists, who are considered ancillary clinical staff in Medicare regulations. Staying current is critical, and CMS provides a weekly Medicare Learning Network newsletter and other helpful resources to assist providers. The resources are publicly available, and pharmacists may sign up to receive weekly announcements regarding rules and resources at the following link: https://www.cms.gov/Outreach-and-Education/Outreach/FFSProvPartProg/Electronic-Mailing-Lists.

Medicare Part A covers hospital, long-term care services, hospice, and certain home health services that occur after an institutional stay. Since beneficiaries contribute to Medicare Part A while employed, once they are eligible for benefits, they incur no additional charges when they enroll in Medicare Part A.

Medicare Part B covers outpatient services, which includes services provided by physicians and other advanced practice practitioners that have Part B provider status, some preventive services, and some homecare services. Medicare beneficiaries are automatically enrolled in Part B when they become eligible for benefits and must opt out if they do not wish to participate and pay the required monthly premium. If a beneficiary does not have existing full retirement or employment health insurance and delays signing up for Medicare Part B beyond when they are first eligible, the beneficiary faces a financial penalty if they enroll at a later time. Most of the reimbursement opportunities for pharmacist patient care services, including those related to telehealth, exist under the Medicare Part B benefit. Payments by CMS for Medicare Part B services are made directly to eligible physicians and nonphysician providers, referred to in CMS regulations as qualified healthcare professionals. As previously noted, pharmacists are not considered healthcare providers under federal healthcare law and are not included in the list of eligible nonphysician providers. Medicare Part B rules published in the physician fee schedule (PFS) and the Hospital Outpatient Prospective Payment System (HOPPS) documents are updated annually at the end of the calendar year.

Medicare Part C is a benefit plan whose structure is based on a managed-care model. CMS outsources the management and design of these plans to approved commercial payers. Each plan, referred to as Medicare Advantage plan, must offer all the benefits under Parts A and B and abide by CMS established rules, but they are free to add more benefits if desired, such as vision, dental, hearing, or prescription drug coverage. Plans may set their own out-of-pocket costs and make additional rules such as requiring primary care to approve referrals for specialists. Unlike Medicare Part B, where the fee for service is paid to the provider, CMS pays the commercial Medicare Part C plan a set amount per member per month. Attached to the payment are required quality measures known as Star Ratings. The plans may receive both financial and program incentives if they can achieve a 4–5 rating on their Star Ratings on a 1–5 scale. Plans with poor ratings in the 1–2 range risk reductions in payment as well as termination from the program. Payers establish their own structure to pay providers for services under the Medicare Advantage plans, generally following processes similar to other benefit plans in their portfolio. Medicare Advantage plans have seen a steady rise over the past 10 years, with over 24 million beneficiaries currently in such plans, which is 36% of all Medicare enrollees.[6] To receive reimbursement for services provided from Medicare Advantage plans, pharmacists need to work with their organizations to ensure their services are included in the organization's agreements with the Medicare Part C contracted commercial payers.

Medicare Part D is the newest Medicare benefit, enacted in 2003 through the Medicare Modernization Act. As with Medicare Part B, beneficiaries contribute to Medicare Part D with monthly premiums and may opt out of this benefit; however, if they do not have acceptable prescription coverage and then decide to opt back in later, they will incur financial penalties. CMS contracts with commercial companies, referred to as Prescription Drug Plans (PDPs), to administer the plan. The PDP is paid a direct subsidy payment by CMS per enrollee with risk adjustments, administrative fees, quality bonuses or penalties, and reinsurance payments for high-cost enrollees. As most pharmacists are aware, this benefit includes medication therapy management (MTM) services, which PDPs fund out of their administrative fees. This benefit provides an opportunity for pharmacists to provide patient care services. Each PDP, within CMS rules, may design how its MTM program is delivered. To obtain reimbursement for Part D MTM services, pharmacists should contract with the PDPs offering benefits within the community or state where they practice; or they may use vendors that contract with payers who develop a network of pharmacists and pharmacies to provide the MTM benefit. Like Part C, Star Ratings based on quality metrics are attached to the payment PDPs receive with similar incentives or penalties based on the star level achieved.

Tool for telehealth pharmacy practice billing: Although it is the PDPs that are required to report on Star Ratings, the responsibility of achieving the ratings is often pushed to the pharmacy. Pharmacists should be aware of these Star Ratings, which may change over time, particularly for Part D. Many of the measures can be positively impacted by leveraging telehealth. For example, one measure associated with medication use is related to medication adherence. Pharmacists can utilize telehealth pharmacy practice to follow up with patients to optimize their adherence. By positively impacting Star Ratings, pharmacies ensure that PDPs will want to continue contracting with them. Part C Star Ratings can also be impacted by leveraging telehealth services to optimize clinical quality measures, such as helping patients control their diabetes.

MEDICARE ADMINISTRATIVE CONTRACTORS (MACs)

Medicare Parts A and B contract with private commercial organizations to assist in administering the benefits. The Medicare Administrative Contractors (MACs) are responsible for enrolling providers into Medicare, processing fee-for-service claims, managing reimbursements, making audits of provider billing, and providing education regarding Medicare rules. MACs also may add interpretation to Medicare billing codes. Historically, these interpretations have significantly affected pharmacists' reimbursement; therefore, it is wise to check with your region's MAC for any additional rules prior to recommending any Medicare billing code for your services. The United States is divided into 12 regions, each with its own MAC contract (**Figure 6.1**). You will note that the same company may have a contract with multiple regions.

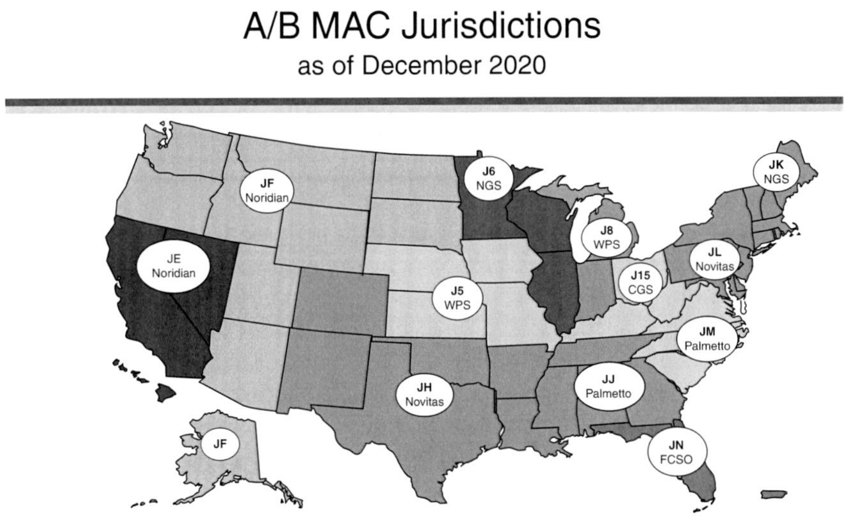

Figure 6.1. CMS MAC contracts per region as of December 2020

Source: FCSO—First Coast Service Options, NGS—National Government Services, WPS—Wisconsin Physician Services https://www.cms.gov/files/document/ab-jurisdiction-map-dec-2020.pdf. Accessed May 18, 2021.

REFERENCES

1. Weaver K. Provider status in the states. *Pharm Times*. 2014;4:41.
2. Weaver KK. Overview of state provider status legislative activity in 2016. *Pharm Today*. 2016;22:68-69.
3. American Medical Association. New research on physicians' patient mix. **www.ama-assn.org/press-center/press-releases/ama-releases-new-research-physicians-patient-mix**. Accessed May 11, 2021.
4. Correspondence with Krystalyn Weaver. National Alliance of State Pharmacy Associations. June 2, 2017.
5. Center for Connected Health Policy, 2020. State Telehealth Laws and Reimbursement Policies Spring 2021. **https://cchp.nyc3.digitaloceanspaces.com/2021/04/Spring2021_ExecutiveSummary.pdf**. Accessed May 11, 2021.
6. Freed M, Damico A, Neuman T. A dozen facts about Medicare Advantage in 2020. Kaiser Family Foundation. 2020; **https://www.kff.org/medicare/issue-brief/a-dozen-facts-about-medicare-advantage-in-2020**. Accessed May 11, 2021.

CHAPTER 7
Regulatory and Financial Considerations of Billing for Telehealth Pharmacy Practice

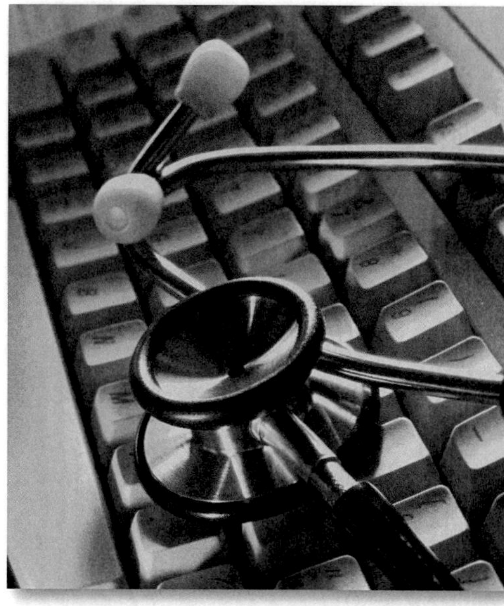

THE LANGUAGE OF HEALTHCARE BILLING

To communicate with those who are responsible for managing, submitting, and paying medical claims, it is beneficial to understand the process, common terms, and general rules utilized. Healthcare fee-for-service billing uses a payment process that employs code sets that describe what service, product, or procedure was provided (Healthcare Common Procedure Coding System [HCPCS] codes); why it was provided (10th revision of the International Statistical Classification of Diseases and Related Health Problems [ICD-10] codes); and who provided it (National Provider Identifier [NPI] number; **Figure 7.1**). A tax identification number (TIN) may be used in place of the NPI number if the claim is being submitted by an organization rather than an individual provider such as a hospital, health system, or medical group. The HCPC code is further adjusted by a factor called relative value units (RVUs) that considers variability in provider cost, value, and liability of the work performed when providing the service being billed.

Healthcare Common Procedure Coding System (HCPCS) Codes

HCPCS codes, often referred to as "hick picks," describe what was provided to the patient by the billing provider and may reflect a service, product, or procedure (**Table 7.1**). There are two levels of HCPCS codes: Level 1, which contains the Current Procedural Terminology (CPT) codes, which have five numeric digits (e.g., 99211), and Level 2 codes, which unlike Level 1 codes, begin with a letter followed by four numeric digits (e.g., G0108). The HCPC Level 1 CPT codes are owned and maintained by the American Medical Association (AMA) and licensed for use by CMS. An AMA standing committee creates, defines, reviews, updates, and distributes the CPT codes. There are three categories of CPT codes, for which only category 1 is used for patient care services. Within category 1 there are six subsections. The subsections of evaluation and management (E&M) and medicine, which contain the MTM codes, are the CPT codes usually used by eligible providers for reimbursement of pharmacist patient care services. Although Medicare does not recognize MTM codes under Medicare Part B, commercial plans may use the MTM codes in Medicare Part C and D if they so choose.

Because not all products and services are included in the AMA CPT codes, CMS created HCPC Level 2 codes. The categories of HCPC Level 2 codes range from A through V. The G codes are used for professional services and provide opportunities for pharmacist reimbursement for services, including several for direct reimbursement of diabetes-related services.

DOI 10.37573/9781585286928.007

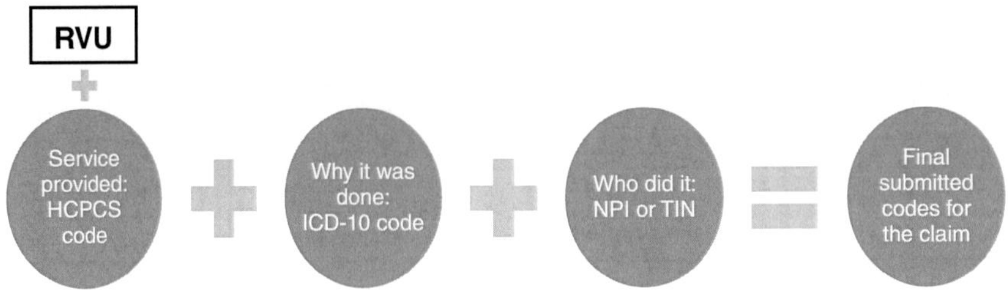

Figure 7.1. Healthcare billing structure

Table 7.1. HCPC Code Categories

Level 1 HCPC CPT Codes	

Category 1
• Evaluation and management (E&M): 99201–99499
  ◦ Example 99211–99215 (established patient codes)
• Anesthesia: 00100–01999; 99100–99150
• Surgery: 10000–69990
• Radiology: 70000–79999
• Pathology and laboratory: 80000–89398
• Medicine: 90281–99099; 99151–99199; 99500–99607
  ◦ Example 99605–99607 MTM codes
	Category 2
	• Supplementary tracking codes that are intended to be used for performance measurement. They are 4-digit numeric codes with an F at the end.
	Category 3
	• Emerging technology temporary codes have a T after the code, designating they are temporary.

Level 2 HCPC Codes	
A Codes: Transportation, medical supplies, miscellaneous, and experimental **B Codes:** Enteral and parenteral therapy **C Codes:** Temporary HOPPS (Hospital Outpatient Prospective Payment System) **D Codes:** Dental procedures **E Codes:** Durable medical equipment (DME) **G Codes:** Temporary procedures and professional services **H Codes:** Rehabilitative services **J Codes:** Drugs administered other than oral method, chemotherapy drugs	**K Codes:** Temporary codes for DME regional carriers **L Codes:** Orthotic/prosthetic procedures **M Codes:** Medical services **P Codes:** Pathology and laboratory **Q Codes:** Temporary codes **R Codes:** Diagnostic radiology services **S Codes:** Private payer codes **T Codes:** State Medicaid agency codes **V Codes:** Vision/hearing services

International Classification of Diseases, 10th Revision (ICD-10) Codes

The "why" a service is provided, or the diagnosis, is identified using a medical classification system termed ICD-10 codes, which are maintained by the World Health Organization under the direction and authority of the United Nations. The 11th Revision, or ICD-11, was released in 2018, with implementation expected to begin January 1, 2022. Besides expanding on new medical conditions and other diagnostic needs, ICD-11 will have improved digital utility linking with other classification and electronic terminologies that offer the promise of facilitating interoperability.

National Provider Identifier (NPI) / Tax Identification Number (TIN)

The provider of a billable service is designated by the NPI number, a 10-digit identification number that all U.S. healthcare providers (pharmacists included) and healthcare organizations can obtain. Administered by CMS, the NPI was created as part of the Health Insurance Portability and Accountability Act of 1996 (HIPAA) for use in electronic transactions of HIPAA information. Healthcare organizations have the option to bill under their TIN. In this situation, the organization must alert CMS to the NPI numbers associated with the submitted billing occurring under their TIN.

Resource-Based Relative Value Scale

The Resource-Based Relative Value Scale (RBRVS) is a payment modifier system created to level the payment due to variation in provider resources and skills associated with CPT billing codes. The practice variations that RBRVS addresses are associated with costs of maintaining a practice (e.g., urban versus rural); level of physician technical skill, required judgment, and stress (e.g., an established patient visit for a neurosurgeon managing a brain tumor vs. a family practitioner managing a common cold); and differences in medical liability costs. Relative value units (RVUs) are added to CPT codes based on a mathematically calculated conversion factor, which is adjusted based on geographic location using the geographic practice cost indexes (GPCI; also referred to as "gypsies"). Because of the geographic adjustments, the reimbursement of any single code will vary across the country. An AMA committee meets several times a year to make RVU value recommendations that CMS reviews and adopts.

Use of Modifiers

Billing modifiers are usually required when delivering telehealth services, most often when using codes that would be utilized during face-to-face encounters. Billing modifiers provide additional information about the service and may be used to help describe why multiple codes are being billed (i.e., using modifier 25 when conducting an Annual Wellness Visit [AWV] the same day a physician sees the patient for a problem-focused visit) or some other nuance to the service provided, such as modality. Similarly, it must be understood whether regulations require each code and/or service to utilize both audio/video technologies or whether other modalities are allowed.

Universal Billing Forms

Billing forms developed by CMS are utilized as the universal forms for submitting bills to Medicare and most other payers of healthcare services. For services reimbursed under Medicare Part A, the paper CMS-1450 form, also called the Universal Billing or UB04 form, is used; the electronic version is called 837I. For services paid under Medicare Part B, the paper CMS-1500 form is the standard form and the 837P form is used for electronic submissions. Instructions for completing the forms may be found on the CMS website.

GENERAL BILLING RULES

To prevent fraud and abuse, CMS has established rules to govern Medicare billing. CMS states that billing charges should be usual, customary, and reasonable; meaning that charges should be the same or similar to other like providers delivering the same medical service within a geographic area. Thus, the charges for your service should be equivalent to what is a typical cost or charge for pharmacists in your area providing the same service. This rule needs to be considered when subcontracting with a provider who will bill your services as incident-to theirs. A second rule is that services should be medically necessary, defined as healthcare services or supplies needed to prevent, diagnose, or treat an illness, injury, condition, disease, or its symptoms meet accepted standards of medicine. When services are referred to a pharmacist, the medical necessity for such a referral in treating the patient's condition should be documented by the referring provider. A third rule is that providers accepting Medicare and Medicaid payment may not discriminate against Medicare and Medicaid patients; for example, they cannot provide a different level of service for Medicare or Medicaid patients versus their service for commercial patients for the same billing code. To avoid risk of Medicare fraud or abuse, unless there exists a specific contract with payers, providers and payers universally follow Medicare rules for submitting bills to request payment for services provided.

TELEHEALTH PHARMACY PRACTICE SPECIFICS

An understanding of billing codes and mechanisms for pharmacists is a necessary foundation for exploring how to appropriately provide and bill for telehealth pharmacy practice services. Similarly, deciphering the CMS guidelines for billing and reimbursement can often be the most challenging task in establishing a sustainable telehealth pharmacy practice service. While CMS is not the only payer of telehealth pharmacy practice services, as mentioned, it often sets the precedent for how other payers will set up their services. It is important to note that in order to get proper reimbursement for telehealth pharmacy practice services, you must understand not only the federal and state regulations, but also the documentation requirements, codes allowed under telehealth, and what services can actually be performed under these codes. The combination of this information becomes the who, what, where, and how of telehealth pharmacy practice delivery and billing.

- *Who*: The who of telehealth regulations refers to which provider or healthcare professional types can bill these services. Medicare originally designated only nine provider types as being allowed to bill telehealth encounters that included Medicare B recognized providers, such as physicians, nurse practitioners, and physician assistants. Since the COVID-19 public health emergency (PHE), all qualified healthcare professionals may bill for services within their scope of practice via telehealth. As a reminder, pharmacists are not a qualified healthcare professional per Medicare rules and regulations. Thus, they cannot directly bill Medicare, but their services may be billed incident-to a physician or Medicare-eligible provider when certain requirements are met.
- *What*: The what of telehealth describes the specific list of services and codes that can be provided via telehealth. Refer to link (updated Aug 2021): https://www.cms.gov/Medicare/Medicare-General-Information/Telehealth/Telehealth-Codes.
- *Where:* The where of telehealth refers to not only where the patient is located but also to the provider. Prior to COVID-19, patients had to be located a specific distance away from the clinic and/or in a healthcare provider shortage area. Likewise, the regulations specified providers must render services from their billing locations. Federal regulations have now waived the location requirements to allow both patients and providers to engage in telehealth visits from their homes. This continues to evolve and may vary between payers and state regulations. Generally, the patient and provider must be physically present in the state in which the provider is licensed. State and commercial payer requirements may vary.
- *How*: The how of telehealth relates to the specific modality of delivery. Whether the visit is audio/video, audio only, asynchronous messaging (such as via a portal), or remote patient monitoring differs in which providers or ancillary team members can perform and bill for each modality. The how may also refer to the platform used and the requirements for each modality.

CHAPTER 8 Tools to Build a Billable Telehealth Pharmacy Practice: Codes and Population Considerations

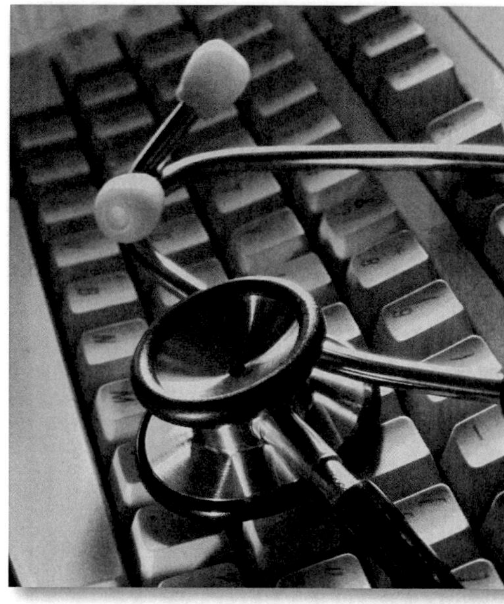

REVENUE-GENERATING OPPORTUNITIES FOR PHARMACISTS

Fee-for-Service

Although alternative payment models (APMs) are increasingly being used as a reimbursement method, fee-for-service (FFS) and use of HCPC codes remain prevalent in most practices. Since Medicare rules are considered the gold standard for medical billing and the accepted method used by most commercial payers, the discussion herein will focus primarily on Medicare billing options and regulations for pharmacist patient care revenue. It is important to note that commercial payers and state Medicaid may not recognize all Medicare codes, or they may include billing codes within their benefit plans not used by Medicare. The billing codes that may apply to your practice require investigation at the local level to determine what is available for payers in your location and patient population. Generating revenue in a FFS model for pharmacists is dependent on the site of practice (i.e., a health system/hospital outpatient clinic, an independent physician or physician group office or clinic, a federally qualified healthcare center, or a community pharmacy). For practice sustainability, it generally requires using as many eligible codes for pharmacist services as are available and appropriate. Although rules and opportunities may differ between practice sites, many also transcend the practice location and are included in the discussion. The codes are summarized in **Table 8.1**.

Incident-to Rules

When pharmacists provide delegated patient care services as auxiliary clinical staff, including pharmacy telehealth practice, a set of rules known as "incident-to" apply for the majority of FFS codes, with some differences based on practice sites that are noted. These rules were created by CMS as a safety mechanism to ensure that the supervising provider is directing the care of the patient, that the delegation of care is appropriate, and that any immediately needed or more complex level of care outside the scope of the ancillary staff is readily available from the supervising provider. As technology has evolved, CMS has relaxed some rules when using available technology advances in communication for certain situations that are noted below.

The incident-to rules must be adhered to when using "incident-to" codes, and they are summarized in **Table 8.2**. Pharmacists as auxiliary personnel may only provide services to established patients from a referring eligible provider. This rule ensures that the delegating provider has created the plan of care for the patient's medical needs and establishes the medical necessity of the referral. A pharmacist would never be the first provider to see a patient in a practice. The delegating provider may only refer patients for billable services

DOI 10.37573/9781585286928.008

Table 8.1. Criteria for Incident-to Services

Rule	Hospital Outpatient Services	Nonhospital Outpatient Services
Service is provided under the direct supervision of an eligible physician or nonphysician practitioner. Defined as within the suite or office space where the service is performed and immediately available to furnish assistance.	General supervision replaces direct supervision	√
Established patient: Patient must be an established patient with the eligible provider. Must have an initial face-to-face visit with the provider where the plan of care is established.	√	√
Service is an integral, though incidental, part of the eligible provider's services.	√	√
Services are commonly rendered without charge or are included as part of the eligible provider's bill.	√	√
Services are of a type that is commonly furnished and appropriate to be provided in a physician's offices or clinic.	√	√
Service must be medically necessary, authorized (authorized practitioner's order), and documented.	√	√
Authorized provider must provide subsequent services at a frequency that reflects active participation in treating the patient and plan of care.	√	√
Financial relationship must exist between the auxiliary personnel and the eligible provider.	Must be an employee, leased employee, or independent contractor	√
Services provided are within the scope of practice for the auxiliary personnel as dictated by the state practice act.	√	√

that they would otherwise provide in their practice. If the provider were not delegating the service, they would be responsible for providing the care needed. The supervising provider must continue to actively manage the plan of care as evidenced by documentation and continued visits with the patient. It would be unacceptable for a patient to have seen only the pharmacist for any extended period of time. An example would be a situation where a chronic anticoagulation patient has only seen the pharmacist for a year of care. The auxiliary clinical staff may only provide services that are within their scope of practice as defined by their state's practice act. As state pharmacy practice acts vary in delineating the patient care services a pharmacist may provide, what is billable by supervising providers for pharmacist services will differ throughout the country.

Supervision of the auxiliary clinic staff is required by the billing provider and differs for certain billing codes and practice sites (see Table 8.2 and the code descriptions below). Certain billing codes require direct supervision, meaning the supervising provider is physically in the suite where the patient care is being provided but does not need to physically be in the visit room. For telehealth pharmacy practice services, direct supervision can be provided virtually, meaning that it is met through immediate accessible audio/video technology. Other billing codes and outpatient services provided and billed under a hospital TIN require general supervision, which is defined as evidence that the supervising provider is directing the plan of care and there is bidirectional sharing and communication of the patient's care plan. For general supervision, there is no requirement of physical accessibility of the supervising provider.

Ancillary clinical staff must be an expense to the billing provider. In the hospital setting, the ancillary staff must be an employee or contracted independent provider. For other settings, the

Table 8.2. Summary of Billing Codes Available for Pharmacist Services Reimbursement

Billing Code Description	Billing Codes	Sites Where Codes May Be Used	"Incident-to Rule" Comments	Telehealth Specifics	Additional Comments
Annual Wellness Visits (AWV)	G0438, G0439	Hospital outpatient Physician offices FQHC	Direct supervision	Can be done audio/video, NOT audio only Requires use of GT or 95 modifier	Vital signs can be waived during public health emergency
Chronic Care Management (CCM) and Complex Chronic Care Management	99490, 99439 99487, 99489	Hospital outpatient Physician offices	General supervision	The codes are intended to be telephonic; however that is not a requirement.	FQHCs have separate codes; see General Care Management
Continuous Glucose Monitoring (CGM)	95249, 95250, 95251	Hospital outpatient Physician offices	Direct supervision	Can be done telephonic with access to data	
Diabetes Self-Management Training (DSMT)	G0108, G0109	Any setting	N/A	Must use audio/video platform or state reason for use of audio only Requires use of 95 modifier	Requires referral from a Medicare-eligible Part B provider and accreditation from ADA or ACDES
Established Patient Evaluation and Management (E/M) codes	99211-99215	Physician offices	Direct supervision	Can be done audio/video, NOT audio only Requires use of GT or 95 modifier	Pharmacist services may only be billed at 99211
General Care Management	G0511	FQHCs only	General supervision		In place of CCM, complex CCM and PCM services in an FQHC
International Normalized Ratio (INR) Monitoring	93792, 93793	Hospital outpatient Physician offices	Direct supervision		
Medicare Diabetes Prevention Program (MDPP)	G9873-G9879, G9880-G9885, G9890, G9891	No requirements	N/A	First visit still in person; others can be telehealth Can restart the series at any time	Requires recognition from the CDC's DPRP
Medication Therapy Management (MTM)	99605, 99606, 99607	No requirements	N/A	Can be done telephonic	Codes not recognized by Medicare
Primary Care Management* (PCM)	G2065, refer to 2022 Physician Fee Schedule for proposed conversion to E/M codes	Physician offices	General supervision	The codes are intended to be telephonic; however that is not a requirement.	FQHCs have separate codes; see General Care Management
Remote Physiologic Monitoring (RPM)	99453, 99457, 99458	Hospital outpatient Physician offices	General supervision		
Transitional Care Management (TCM)	99495,99496	Hospital outpatient Physician offices FQHC	General supervision		Requires physician visit at 7 or 14 days to bill

rules are not as specific, stating that the ancillary clinical staff must be an expense to the billing provider through a financial relationship. A practice site may not bill for pharmacist services without reasonable and customary remuneration to the pharmacist for their services.

Hospital or Health-System Billing ("Facility Fee" Billing) Codes: APC 4012 with G-0463

Payment rules for hospital outpatient services are governed by the Hospital Outpatient Prospective Payment System (HOPPS); they differ in payment for the same services provided in independent physician offices and clinics. Facility costs such as electricity and janitorial services are a separate charge from services in the hospital reimbursement structure. In the same manner, facility costs in HOPPS are not woven into the code reimbursement amounts, as it is for the Physician Fee Schedule. When outpatient services are provided and billed under the hospital's TIN, a professional fee is billed by the eligible Medicare provider, and a "facility fee" is paid to the hospital for the facility costs of providing the service to a beneficiary. Pharmacist services in this setting are billed as a facility fee charge incident-to with general supervision by an eligible Medicare Part B provider by the hospital. Similar to how inpatient service payments are grouped, outpatient patient care service payment is grouped together into ambulatory payment classifications (APCs), with the addition of a clinical services HCPC code. Patient care services provided by pharmacists in the hospital outpatient setting are billed under APC code 4012 and HCPC II code G-0463. These codes are subject to "incident-to rules" and as of 2020 require general supervision by the supervising provider.

CPT EVALUATION AND MANAGEMENT (E/M) CODES

Patient care in the ambulatory setting is best represented by the evaluation and management (E/M) codes. These codes describe the level and complexity of medical evaluation and management of a patient by a provider during an ambulatory visit. When utilized for a billable interaction, the work provided should include three major components of care: history, examination, and medical decision making.[1] Several codes (CMM, PCM) are exceptions to this rule, in that time spent in the visit determines the code chosen for reimbursement. CMS defines medical decision making as the complexity of establishing a diagnosis and/or selecting a management option.[1] Documentation of services provided must demonstrate the required elements of the E/M code being used for billing. Guidance for the element requirements is outlined in the specifications created by the AMA for the CPT codes and in the annual CMS Physician Fee Schedule rulings. The following codes are available E/M codes that may include pharmacist patient care services. All billed codes must be submitted by a supervising provider and meet incident-to rules. As mentioned, supervision requirements and additional details needed for billing can be different for telehealth codes.

Established Patient (99211-99215)

Established patient codes are the main codes used for patient visits in the ambulatory physician office or clinic setting and are recognized by all payers. The codes may also be used in the health system or hospital setting for Medicare billing when ambulatory services are billed under a physician or medical provider group NPI and not the hospital TIN. Hospitals and health systems may choose to incorporate their medical groups and bill established patient codes as a physician group and not under the hospital TIN in lieu of a facility fee. A rationale for doing so allows the medical group to be for profit and the hospital to remain nonprofit. Established patient codes require direct supervision when used as incident-to services.

For incident-to services, an established patient is defined as a patient initially seen by the referring physician within the previous three years for the same problems for which you as the ambulatory pharmacist (i.e., auxiliary clinical staff) will be providing services. The code used to describe the billable interaction is determined by the visit's level of complexity or the time spent with the patient for coordinating care or education. CMS for 2021 is adopting new E/M documentation requirements for new and established patients developed by the AMA. An advantage of the new guidance is that it improves the efficiency of necessary documentation and reduces redundancy.[2] A negative for pharmacists is that the AMA document states that incident-to services by auxiliary personnel cannot be billed higher than 99211 and that time-based coding may only be used by providers who can independently bill. Until this 2021 CMS ruling, the level for which services provided by pharmacists as auxiliary personnel should be billed had been unclear, resulting in varied interpretations by both MACs and compliance officers as to whether higher codes than 99211 may be used. In the 2021 PFS, CMS states that although they recognize that other payers may pay pharmacists directly for patient care services, under Medicare, pharmacists are not among the qualified healthcare providers that may furnish services billed at 99212-5. In addition, CMS stated that time-based billing cannot be billed as "incident-to."[3] As of January 1, 2021, pharmacist services billed to Medicare as "incident-to" established patient visits were limited to the 99211 level. Commercial payers and state Medicaid may opt to utilize all code levels for incident-to established patients for delegated pharmacist services. Generally, as Medicare is the gold standard in healthcare reimbursement, other payers tend to follow CMS's rules.

Telehealth Specifics

In general, *most* services provided by pharmacists are eligible for 99211 billing, such as those rendered under collaborative drug therapy management protocols and collaborative practice agreements. The 99211 code may also be billed utilizing audio/video visits via telehealth. These visits generally require the use of a GT (via interactive audio and video telecommunications) or a 95 modifier to show they were completed via telehealth versus in person.

While typical disease management visits such as diabetes and hypertension would be reimbursed under this model, it is always important to check state regulations as well for any exclusions for telehealth. For example, many states have regulations regarding face-to-face requirements for patients receiving opioid or controlled substance prescriptions, but these have traditionally excluded telehealth as a way to complete these visits. In the current COVID-19 public health emergency, many states have waived the in-person requirement, but this highlights the need to ensure that even if the code being billed is covered via telehealth, you are also meeting requirements for the particular service under this code.

Chronic Care Management—CCM (99490, G99439) or Complex Chronic Care Management—Complex CCM (99487, 99489)

CCM and complex CCM are available billing codes for hospitals or health systems' outpatient services and medical offices.[4] These codes are designed for services delegated to auxiliary personnel. Both types of CCM services may be provided under general supervision, which allows the service to be provided at a different site than the supervising provider. Pharmacists may be in a location other than where the supervising provider practices, including pharmacies. Beneficiaries qualify for CCM if they have two or more of any type of chronic condition that will last at least 12 months, or until the patient's death; and the condition places the patient at significant risk of death, acute exacerbation, decompensation, or functional decline. Complex CCM is intended for the category of patients requiring moderate- or high-complexity medical decision making, with evidence of the complexity documented. CCM codes may be non-face-to-face; therefore, services may be provided via any telehealth modality, including phones.

CCM has a set of rules that the healthcare team must adhere to when providing and billing for this service, including the following:

- Patient consent
- The referring provider's initiating face-to-face patient visit
    - During the public health emergency, this requirement was waived and can be completed telephonically

- 24/7 access to team members
- Electronic and shared comprehensive care plan and ongoing assessment, as appropriate for the patient
- Enhanced continuity with community services

The CCM codes are billed monthly and may only be submitted by one provider per patient. However, services can be provided by multiple clinical staff of the billing provider. The code 99490 is billed for the first 20 minutes of services, with the option for two additional 20-minute units (code G2058) of services if needed per month. Complex CCM is billed with code 99487 for the first 60 minutes of clinical staff time; if an additional 30 minutes is needed, CPT code 99489 is used. For more details, visit CMS's Medical Learning Network for up-to-date guidance material (CMS Chronic Care Management).

Primary Care Management*—PCM (G2065)

PCM follows CCM rules and regulations. Unlike CCM, PCM is intended for a single high-risk disease or complex condition expected to last at least 3 months to 1 year where the condition may have led to a recent hospitalization and/or may have placed the patient at significant risk of death, acute exacerbation or decompensation, or functional decline. PCM is available for physician offices or clinics. CMS intends PCM to be used for a complex condition that requires management by a more specialized practitioner than primary care. The specialist would stabilize the condition and then return care to primary care. CMS, however, places no restrictions on which specialty may use the codes and acknowledges that primary care may also provide the service and use the code.

PCM may be billed by more than one practitioner. However, the same practitioner cannot bill CCM with PCM. CMS created two initial codes for PCM. G2064 is to be used when PCM services are provided by an eligible Medicare provider, and G2065 is to be used when clinical staff (i.e., pharmacists) under incident-to rules and general supervision provide the service. Like CCM, PCM may be provided under general supervision.

Transitional Care Management—TCM (99495, 99496)

Like CCM, TCM codes are available for payment in hospitals or health systems, medical offices, and federally qualified health centers.[5] This Medicare benefit is intended to reduce 30-day rehospitalization by reimbursing for care management and care coordination after a discharge from an institution (inpatient hospital, rehabilitation and psychiatric institutions, observational inpatient stays of less than 48 hours, skilled nursing facility) to the community. The billable services have two components: a telephonic portion that permits auxiliary clinical staff to perform a set of services under incident-to rules and general supervision; and a face-to-face visit that must be provided by a Medicare-eligible billing provider.

The telephonic component requires interactive communication with the patient or caregiver within two business days of discharge. This may be done by the billing provider or licensed clinical staff within their state scope of practice under incident-to rules and general supervision. Telephone, email, or text messaging are all acceptable for this interaction. CMS does not specify that the required elements of this visit other than care management and coordination should occur.

The face-to-face component must be furnished by the billing provider either within 7 days for a patient requiring high-complexity medical decision making using the 99496 code or within 14 days for less complex patients using the 99495 code. As with CCM, only one provider may bill for TCM services, and the charge may only be used once within a 30-day period regardless of the number of admissions or discharges during that period. More details on utilizing this code may be found in the CMS MLN Newsletter for TCM services.

---

*Note for 2022: CMS is proposing to change the G code to a 99X24 and a 99X25 code. Final decision will be around 12/1/2021.

Remote Physiologic Monitoring—RPM (99453, 99457, 99458)

RPM codes are available for hospital, health-system outpatient and physician offices, or clinics.[2] RPM codes pay for the collection and analysis of patient physiologic data collected through a remote device, where the device is used to develop and manage a treatment plan related to a chronic and/or acute health illness or condition. The device (e.g., weight scales, blood pressure monitors, pulse oximeters) must meet the Food and Drug Administration (FDA) definition of a medical device and should automatically upload patient physiologic data through digital means and not be data that are patient self-recorded and/or self-reported. Services may only be billed for established patients.

Auxiliary clinical staff (e.g., pharmacists) may provide setup and monitoring of RPM services incident-to a Medicare-qualified provider under general supervision. The initial setup and patient education on use of the equipment may be provided and billed once using code 99453. Monitoring of daily transmissions or programmed alerts received from the patient's device may be billed using code 99454 submitted every 30 days and must have at least 16 days of data. Auxiliary clinical staff may provide management of therapy related to remote physiologic monitoring through interactive communication with the patient or their caregiver for at least 20 minutes during the calendar month to bill code 99457. An add-on code of 99458 is available for each additional 20 minutes as needed. Interactive communication is defined as real-time synchronous two-way audio interaction (i.e., phone) that is capable of being enhanced with video or other kinds of data transmission. It should be noted that the physiologic data, billed as code 99091, may only be interpreted by an eligible Medicare provider.

Telehealth Specifics

Chronic or Complex Management (CCM), Remote Physiologic Monitoring (RPM), Principal Care Management (PCM), and the pharmacist's role in Transitional Care Management (TCM) have always been allowed via telephonic means. With primary care and pharmacist-specific revenue decreasing with fewer in-person visits, renewed interest and understanding of CCM, RPM, and PCM have occurred. No additional regulations beyond those discussed previously are required to utilize these through telehealth means as these are not considered telehealth codes.

CPT MEDICINE CODES

Continuous Glucose Monitoring—CGM (95249, 95250, 95251)

CGM is available for payment in hospital/health-system ambulatory care practices and physician offices and requires direct supervision incident-to an eligible Medicare provider. CGM is a glucose monitoring modality available to patients with diabetes who require frequent testing, dosing of their insulin, and adjustment of their therapeutic regimen. Because CMS has deferred CGM regulations to the MACs, variation in requirements may exist between MACs, and MAC regulations should be reviewed prior to utilizing the codes.

There are two types of CGMs: (1) one for personal use where interstitial glucose level data are presented directly to the patient for real-time self-management and (2) one for professional-use CGMs where data are transmitted for interpretation by a healthcare provider. Personal-use CGMs may be limited due to their cost. Most payers provide coverage for professional-use CGMs. For personal-use CGMs, CPT code 95249 may be billed once for education and training of a personal-use CGM. For professional-use CGMs, CPT code 95250 may be billed monthly for CGM sensor placement or removal and supplying equipment, calibration, printout of recording, and patient training. CPT code 95251 may be billed monthly for analysis, interpretation, and reporting of at least 72 hours of glucose data for either personal- or professional-CGM use.

Telehealth Specifics

Current regulations do not require the face-to-face component in order to bill for CGM services outside of device placement. Similarly, local coverage determinations for requirements for obtaining a CGM device have been waived during the public health emergency, allowing greater access for patients. Providers can then utilize online portals or patient-provided uploads for CGM interpretation and glucose management.

International Normalized Ratio Monitoring—INR (93792, 93793)

INR monitoring codes are available for hospital/health-system outpatient and physician office billing for clinical staff under direct supervision by a physician or other qualified healthcare professional. CPT code 93792 is for billing patients or caregiver training for initiation of home INR monitoring; it includes use and care of the INR monitor, obtaining a blood sample, instructions for reporting home INR test results, and documentation of the patient's or caregiver's ability to perform testing and report results. CPT code 93793 is for billing review and interpretation or an INR and anticoagulant management for a patient taking warfarin obtained in the home, office, or lab. It therefore includes telephonic monitoring. Documentation should include patient instructions, dosage adjustment (as needed), and scheduling of additional test(s).[6] The reimbursement rate for this code is lower than the established patient code 99211 and thus is less commonly used.

Medication Therapy Management Codes—MTM (99605, 99606, 99607)

Medicare does not recognize MTM codes for direct reimbursement to a provider in any of its benefit plans. The MTM codes may be available for reimbursement under state Medicaid, from PDPs in executing the Medicare Part D MTM requirements and some commercial payers. MTM codes are time based, with code 99605 used for the initial 15 minutes of a face-to-face visit with a new patient. Code 99606 bills for the initial 15 minutes of a face-to-face visit with an established patient, and 99607, as an add-on code for each additional 15 minutes for either a new or an established patient.

While CPT definition of MTM codes is face-to-face, these codes have been utilized via telephonic interactions for several years, and current telehealth regulatory changes did not affect the payment or delivery of these codes. Current reimbursement for these codes remains through Medicare Part D or other direct contracted plans.

HCPCS LEVEL II G CODES

Annual Wellness Visits—AWV (G0438, G0439)

AWV codes are available for payment in hospitals or health systems, medical offices, and federally qualified healthcare centers. The AWV is a benefit meant to focus on wellness and disease prevention, and thus, like other preventive services from CMS, it does not have an associated copay. Three visit types are included in the benefit, of which only two may be provided by ancillary licensed clinical staff under direct supervision of the eligible billing provider. The first service under the AWV benefit is the IPPE—the initial preventive physical examination (G0402 code)—that may only be provided by an eligible Medicare Part B provider. This visit is also referred to as the "Welcome to Medicare" visit. The initial Annual Wellness Visit (G0438) is conducted one year later; it is billed only once and may be provided by ancillary clinical staff. Thereafter, an AWV with clinical staff may occur each year and is billed under code G0439. Each code has an associated set of screenings and services that must be provided to bill the code. Details for the AWV requirements may be found on the CMS Medical Learning Network website.[7]

Telehealth Specifics

AWVs are also allowed to be conducted via audio/video two-way communication with the patient; audio only visits are not considered billable. Similar to established patient codes, a GT or 95 modifier is required when submitting claims. All elements of the AWV, whether initial or subsequent, must be met with the potential exception of the vitals component. Patients can self-report height, weight, and blood pressure if able. Under current circumstances, it is also acceptable to waive the vitals component with the additional documentation of "unable to obtain due to COVID-19 public health emergency."

Although pharmacists are unable to perform the initial preventive physical exam (IPPE-G0402), it is important to note that this exam is also not allowable via telehealth.

General Care Management for FQHCs Only (G0511)

FQHCs are eligible to bill for CCM, complex CCM, and PCM services. For FQHCs the codes 99490, 99487, and G2065 are collapsed into one code, G0511, and submitted by the FQHC when any of these services are provided.

Diabetes Self-Management Training—DSMT (G0108, G0109)

DSMT is available for billing by any provider in any setting, including pharmacists practicing within their state scope of practice. Requirements are that the service must be initiated by an order from a Medicare-Qualified Provider who is managing the patient's diabetes stating there is a medical need for DSMT, and the DSMT program must have accreditation from either the Association of Diabetes Care and Education Specialists (ADCES) or the American Diabetes Association (ADA). A list of diabetes topics must be included in the curriculum, and the education must be provided within a set education visit timeframe and frequency over a 12-month period. The education may be provided individually (G0108) or to a group of patients with diabetes (G0109), with each method having its own rules for length and frequency of instruction. Additional details on DSMT regulations may be found on the Government Publication Office website.[8]

Telehealth Specifics

Accredited DSMT programs eligible to directly bill Medicare, including pharmacists providing services within these programs, can provide services via telehealth in any healthcare setting. Regulations specify that audio/video communication should be used if at all possible. In addition, if audio only is utilized for services, reason for use must be clearly documented. Use of location modifier 95 is also required for use during these visits. Programs originating out of an outpatient hospital site may still bill for services under the NPI and TIN. Visits can occur via telehealth for both new and established patients.

Medicare Diabetes Prevention Program—MDPP (G9873-G9879, G9880-G9885, G9890, G9891)

MDPP is a service based on structured and evidence-based interventions designed to prevent the onset of type 2 diabetes in Medicare beneficiaries identified with prediabetes. MDPP services are provided by a "coach" who must have an NPI number and must have attained recognition through the Diabetes Prevention Recognition Program (DPRP) from the CDC. The DPRP entails training, reviewing, and completing the CDC's standards and procedure requirements.[9] Providers of this service are from a wide range of background practice sites that include health clubs, health systems, public health organizations, physician offices, and pharmacies. MDPP includes a set of core sessions over the first 6 months, followed by ongoing maintenance sessions for an additional 18 months. The list of codes reflects the different sessions and required documentation. MDPP providers submit claims through the usual Medicare Part B processes, with payments made based on beneficiary attendance and weight loss of 5% from baseline for the first 6 months and 9% from baseline at the completion of the program.

Telehealth Specifics

Providers of MDPP as of March 1, 2020 may provide services virtually. Of note, certain requirements, such as the first session requiring in-person attendance, are still in effect. While some in-person requirements remain, participants whose sessions have been disrupted by the pandemic are now able to start a program over or resume it at a later date. Previously, this had been a once in a lifetime benefit.

SUMMARY OF FEE-FOR-SERVICE BILLING

Presented in this chapter is a small fraction of the available codes used by providers for the services and procedures presently in healthcare delivery. The codes discussed are those where CMS specifically states that services may be delegated to auxiliary personnel or clinical staff to perform under supervision; or codes that CMS allows pharmacists to bill directly as providers. Other existing codes may be used by eligible Medicare providers where the provider is conducting the visit and the pharmacist is participating as clinical staff. These codes were not reviewed as they are billing mainly for the eligible provider's service. Clinical staff is considered a participant. In such situations, the billing provider must adhere to the code requirements in providing the service in conjunction with their staff. Billing is key for financial sustainability. The available codes have variable reimbursement rates that are impacted by location. To determine the current rate of payment for a billing code from Medicare to physician offices (based on location), it is best to access the Physician Fee Schedule Lookup tool: https://www.cms.gov/Medicare/Medicare-Fee-for-Service-Payment/PFSlookup. To obtain payment information for Medicare hospital outpatient, FQHCs, commercial payers, and state Medicaid, it is more challenging and best to work with your compliance officer for this information.

SUMMARY OF TELEHEALTH PHARMACY PRACTICE BILLING TOOLS

This information can be complex, and pharmacists who are delivering telehealth services must be kept informed of, and keep up-to-date with, the ever-evolving details. Upon becoming familiar with these concepts, pharmacists must then be prepared to implement and operationalize telehealth and billing for telehealth pharmacy practice services, which includes ongoing quality control. Many tools need to be included in any pharmacy practice's toolkit to build a practice that optimizes telehealth for billing and reimbursement.

Several key components are important to ensure that billing and regulatory requirements are satisfied, while continuing to guarantee practice efficiency. These should be considered in addition to the concepts discussed in Section 2: Telehealth Pharmacy Practice Workflows. Recognizing supervision and audio/video platform requirements, identifying support and billing staff, and customizing the implementation of telehealth to the specific practice site are among the important considerations. Further, understanding state-specific billing rules and available opportunities is vital to guide development of the telehealth practice.

SUPERVISION OF PHARMACIST TELEHEALTH BILLING

As described previously, a variety of methods are available to carry out telehealth pharmacy practice patient care services, including live video, store-and-forward, remote patient monitoring, and care via email, telephone, and fax. Live video is the most predominantly reimbursed form of telehealth across the nation. Every state offers some type of live video reimbursement in its Medicaid program. There is variability, however, in how the reimbursement is done and for what services (e.g., behavioral health only in New Jersey vs. a wide variety of specialties in California). There are limitations on the types of services that can be delivered and reimbursed via live video, as well as types of providers. The "originating site" refers to the location of the patient, and some states have restrictions on this too.[10] Depending on the service provided, there may also be requirements for pharmacist supervision. Failure to meet these supervision requirements can result in loss of payment in the event of auditing. Pharmacists should ask themselves, What needs to be in place to ensure that supervision requirements are met? The answer will depend on the type of telehealth delivery method as well as the specific service being provided. It is important to determine whether direct or general supervision is required for the service being provided, summarized in Tables 8.1 and 8.2. The COVID-19 pandemic led CMS to allow for a provision that virtual, real-time audio/video technology may be used to satisfy the requirement for direct supervision.[11] By definition, general supervision does not require physical accessibility to the supervising provider, so telehealth methods are therefore an acceptable means of providing care.

To satisfy direct supervision via telehealth, it is important for pharmacists to develop a plan with their physician colleagues. This plan may involve changes to workflows to allow for a method for the physician to be accessible when needed, and also ensure that contact information is available for both the pharmacist and physician colleagues, along with up-to-date work schedules.

Audio/Video Platform Considerations

When planning for implementation of telehealth pharmacy practice services, privacy and security standards must be considered, and ensuring that HIPAA rules are followed is a necessity. The Department of Health and Human Services Office for Civil Rights (OCR) states that healthcare providers must ensure that telehealth is conducted privately. This generally means that the service is delivered by the healthcare professional in a clinic or office connected to a patient in their home or at another site. OCR specifies that patients should not participate in telehealth pharmacy practice visits in a public setting unless consent is provided by the patient or "exigent" circumstances exist. If it is not possible to provide telehealth pharmacy practice services in a private setting, OCR recommends that healthcare professionals continue to abide by HIPAA guidelines in order to minimize any disclosure of protected health information (PHI). Examples can include using lowered voices, avoiding use of a speakerphone, or recommending that the patients position themselves in a location at a reasonable distance from others, especially when discussing PHI.[12]

When delivering telehealth pharmacy practice via live video, the platform used must be "non-public facing." This means that the platform "allows only the intended parties to participate in the communication."[13] Acceptable non-public-facing platforms include Webex, Doximity, Apple FaceTime, Facebook Messenger video chat, Google Hangouts video, Whatsapp video chat, Zoom, or Skype. These platforms typically utilize end-to-end encryption, which allows only an individual and the person with whom the individual is communicating to see and hear what is communicated. Unacceptable platforms that would not be considered nonpublic facing would be those that allow wide access to communication or public, such as a "livestreaming" service. Examples include TikTok, Facebook Live, Twitch, or any public online chat room.

Support Staff Considerations

Meeting with your practice site's billing and/or coding staff (or meeting with your local clinic's staff if practicing in a community pharmacy) can prove vital to ensure that all required elements and information are being properly documented for any telehealth services, as well as to confirm that the appropriate billing codes and modifiers are being submitted. Leveraging registration and nursing staff, pharmacy technicians, and learners can also enhance efficiency when delivering services via telehealth. Examples can include utilizing registration staff to help schedule video visits and provide appropriate login information for patients, nursing staff to start up video visits and collect patient intake information, including vitals (if applicable) and alert you when the patient is ready to be seen ("virtual rooming"), and using pharmacy technicians and learners to perform appropriate delegated tasks such as medication reconciliation.

Monitoring Telehealth Billing Quality

In addition to meeting with billing staff to prepare for compliance with telehealth billing regulations, it is also important to monitor the quality of the telehealth billing process. This can be done by tracking reimbursement through the billing reports generated and by meeting regularly with billing and financial administration to identify problems with billing as well as new opportunities. It is also important to consider continuous review of the cost of telehealth technology, including the platforms used to deliver video visits.

REFERENCES

1. Centers for Medicare and Medicaid. Medical Learning Network. Evaluation and Management Services Guide. January 2020 **https://www.cms.gov/outreach-and-education/medicare-learning-network-mln/mlnproducts/downloads/eval-mgmt-serv-guide-icn006764.pdf**. Accessed May 13, 2021.
2. American Medical Association. CPT® Evaluation and Management (E/M) Office or Other Outpatient (99202-99215) and Prolonged Services (99354, 99355, 99356, 99417) Code and Guideline Changes. 2021. **https://www.ama-assn.org/system/files/2019-06/cpt-office-prolonged-svs-code-changes.pdf**. Accessed May 13, 2021.
3. Center for Medicare and Medicaid Services. Medicare Program; CY 2021 Payment Policies under the Physician Fee Schedule and Other Changes to Part B Payment Policies; Medicare Shared Savings Program Requirements; Medicaid Promoting Interoperability Program Requirements for Eligible Professionals; Quality Payment Program; Coverage of Opioid Use Disorder Services Furnished by Opioid Treatment Programs; Medicare Enrollment of Opioid Treatment Programs; Electronic Prescribing for Controlled Substances for a Covered Part D Drug; Payment for Office/Outpatient Evaluation and Management Services; Hospital IQR Program; Establish New Code Categories; Medicare Diabetes Prevention Program (MDPP) Expanded Model Emergency Policy; Coding and Payment for Virtual Check-in Services Interim Final Rule Policy; Coding and Payment for Personal Protective Equipment (PPE) Interim Final Rule Policy; Regulatory Revisions in Response to the Public Health Emergency (PHE) for COVID-19; and Finalization of Certain Provisions from the March 31st, May 8th and September 2nd Interim Final Rules in Response to the PHE for COVID-19. Federal Register, December 28, 2020.
4. Centers for Medicare and Medicaid Services. Medicare Learning Network: Chronic Care Management Services. 2019. **https://www.cms.gov/outreach-and-education/medicare-learning-network-mln/mlnproducts/downloads/chroniccaremanagement.pdf**. Accessed May 13, 2021.
5. Centers for Medicare and Medicaid Services. Medicare Learning Network: Transitional Care Management. **https://www.cms.gov/Outreach-and-Education/Medicare-Learning-Network-MLN/MLNProducts/Downloads/Transitional-Care-Management-Services-Fact-Sheet-ICN908628.pdf**. Accessed May 18, 2021.
6. Centers for Medicare and Medicaid Services. Medicare Program; Revisions to Payment Policies Under the Physician Fee Schedule and Other Revisions to Part B for CY 2018; Medicare Shared Savings Program Requirements; and Medicare Diabetes Prevention Program. *Federal Register*. 2017. **https://www.federalregister.gov/documents/2017/11/15/2017-23953/medicare-program-revisions-to-payment-policies-under-the-physician-fee-schedule-and-other-revisions**. Accessed May 13, 2021.
7. Centers for Medicare and Medicaid Services. Medicare Learning Network: Annual Wellness Visits. **https://www.cms.gov/Outreach-and-Education/Medicare-Learning-Network-MLN/MLNProducts/preventive-services/medicare-wellness-visits.html**. Accessed May 13, 2021.
8. U.S. Government Publishing Office (GPO). Outpatient Diabetes Self-Management Training and Diabetes Outcome Measurements. **https://www.ecfr.gov/cgi-bin/text-idx?SID=35fab7def9bb9c937d3af534774269df&mc=true&node=sp42.2.410.h&rgn=div6**. Accessed May 13, 2021.
9. Centers for Disease Control. Centers for Disease Control and Prevention Diabetes Prevention Recognition Program Standards and Operating Procedures. March 2018. **https://www.cdc.gov/diabetes/prevention/pdf/dprp-standards.pdf**. Accessed May 13, 2021.
10. CMS. National health expenditures 2019 highlights. **https://www.cms.gov/files/document/highlights.pdf**. Accessed May 13, 2021.
11. U.S. Department of Health & Human Services Office for Civil Rights. Where can health care providers conduct telehealth? March 2020. **https://www.hhs.gov/hipaa/for-professionals/faq/3021/where-can-health-care-providers-conduct-telehealth/index.html**. Accessed May 13, 2021.
12. U.S. Department of Health & Human Services Office for Civil Rights. What is a "non-public facing" remote communication product? April 2020. **https://www.hhs.gov/hipaa/for-professionals/faq/3024/what-is-a-non-public-facing-remote-communication-product/index.html**. Accessed May 13, 2021.
13. Agency for Healthcare Research and Quality. Telehealth: Mapping the Evidence for Patient Outcomes from Systematic Reviews. June 2016. Telehealth: Mapping the Evidence for Patient Outcomes from Systematic Reviews (ahrq.gov).

CHAPTER 9
Integrating the Billing Strategies Alternative to Fee-for-Service

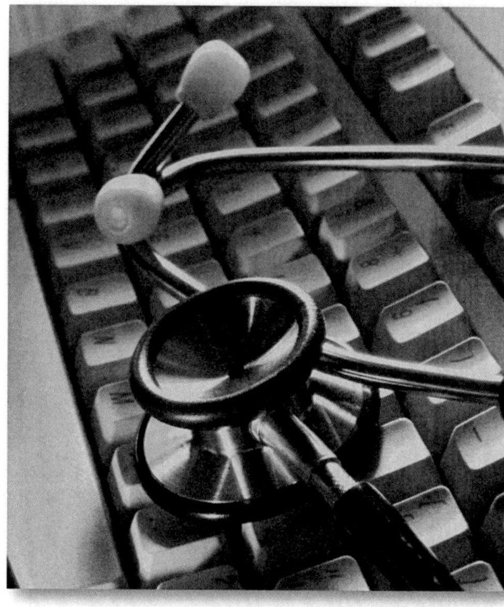

VALUE-BASED PAYMENTS

Unlike fee-for-service where payment occurs by performing an action in caring for a patient, value-based payments pay for the result of the totality of numerous actions delivered in the care of a patient or population. If health improvements occur, providers are rewarded; if not, the providers may be penalized. In healthcare, the usual economic forces where a poor product or service results in declining purchases do not operate as one would expect. This occurs because of healthcare's complex and opaque nature, and those who receive care do not directly pay for the care or in some benefit plans they are restricted in their ability to choose their providers. A situation is created in which a poor-quality service is paid the same amount as an identical service provided with high quality. These dynamics have contributed to the current circumstances facing healthcare in the United States: escalating and unsustainable healthcare costs, and quality of care when compared to other industrialized countries remains at the bottom of the list.[1,2] Waste in our current system, which provides zero value, is estimated at $3,500 per person, or one-third of what is spent on healthcare per person in the United States.[3]

Clearly, a need for change is evident; thus, payers, organizations, and providers are pursuing new and innovative alternative payment models that reward value of services and quality of care. To understand payment based on value, it is necessary to know what value means to the stakeholders involved. A definition proposed by M. E. Porter, a Harvard economist, is the value definition most widely used.[4] Porter states that value refers to outcomes achieved that are important to a patient and specific to the full spectrum of a medical condition per total dollars spent. Value is derived when the maximum health benefit is achieved at the lowest cost. Three main pathways exist to achieve this goal:

1. Improving the benefit of care is greater than any increase in the cost of that care.
2. Decreasing the cost of care without jeopardizing the benefits of that care.
3. Improving benefits of care while decreasing its cost.

VALUE-BASED PAYMENT (VBP) MODELS

Although programs paying for quality began in the 1990s, it was the Affordable Care Act (ACA), passed in 2010, that gave birth to many emerging models. Presently, there exists a spectrum of VBP models that span from quality payment built upon the existing fee-for-service model to payment based on how well a population's health improves. Summarized below are the more prevalent models. Although not universal, all models have examples of pharmacist-provided patient care contributing to a model's value in providing care.

DOI 10.37573/9781585286928.009

Pay for Performance (P4P)

The most common payment model is P4P, which is built on fee-for-service architecture. Providers bill and are paid for services under fee-for-service but have the additional requirement of meeting certain preestablished measures intended to improve the quality and efficiency of care. Payment models vary in that some providers are paid just to report; others have incentive payments if measure benchmarks are met or exceeded. If quality benchmarks are not achieved, for some models there are no consequences other than not receiving the financial incentives; other models incur financial penalties or risk being dropped from the provider network. An advantage of P4P is the ability to measure distinct aspects of care such as blood pressure reduction. It is more challenging to measure holistic outcomes of care compared to other VBP models.

Patient-Centered Medical Home

Patient-Centered Medical Home (PCMH) is a model of care delivery that is also a form of VBP because its five principles of comprehensive care, patient-centered care, coordinated care, accessible services, and quality and safety are considered foundational to achieve value. Providers may acquire a recognition for meeting PCMH standards through accreditation organizations and may be rewarded by certain payers with additional payment or reimbursement.

Accountable Care Organizations

Accountable Care Organizations (ACOs), like PCMH, are a delivery and payment model formed by groups of organizations (hospitals, long-term care facilities, etc.) and healthcare providers (physicians, pharmacists, social workers, etc.) for the purpose of providing highly coordinated and quality care to an attributed population. The premise is that waste will be reduced through intense coordination and focus on quality under a unified structure. ACOs assume the overall accountability of care and costs for the enrolled patients. There are numerous models under the ACO umbrella. ACO models are found in Medicare, Medicaid, and with commercial payers. Central to their structure are the effort to achieve set quality metrics and the concept of positive and negative risk-sharing. A one-sided risk model is one in which the payer and the ACO, based on the ACO's financial performance, share any positive savings that occur. A two-sided risk model is one in which both the payer and the ACO share either positive financial rewards or negative financial losses based on the ACOs' performance.

Clinical Episode or Bundled Payments

Clinical episode or bundled payments address healthcare situations that are episodes of care versus chronic care. The episodes involve multiple providers and settings in care of conditions that have a start and an end; where coordination and managing quality and cost have potential to provide value (e.g., joint replacement, maternity care, myocardial infarction). The model is intended to provide flexibility to healthcare providers to determine what services and resources are needed for the episode to achieve the greatest value. A single comprehensive payment is made to the provider group delivering the services, often with risk sharing as part of the agreement.

Global Payments

Global payments are examples of a mature VBP model, and for many proponents they are the goal for healthcare payment. This model payment is twofold: a fixed per-patient fee is paid to the provider intended to cover the total cost of care for patient services during a set time interval and a payment based on value as described by Porter. The payment structure is provided as payment per patient per month or per year. Providers drive the scope of services needed to achieve the outcomes desired. The incentive is to deliver excellent and efficient patient care to maximize the payment provided. Success is predicated on having the organizational competencies and infrastructure to intensively manage care on both the patient and the population levels.

VALUE-BASED PAYMENT AND PHARMACIST PATIENT CARE SERVICES

To achieve value in patient care and financially sustain healthcare delivery, a team model is essential to provide the necessary services in an efficient and coordinated manner. Medications are the primary therapeutic tool in healthcare, with medication prescriptions included in 75% of primary care visits.[5] Medications are also a significant healthcare problem, causing significant morbidity and mortality and resulting in healthcare costs of $528 billion annually.[6] Thus, medication management services, optimally provided by pharmacists, are integral to VBP models to achieve a goal of overall improvement of health in patients and populations. For medication management, it would make sense that pharmacists, based on their training and knowledge, would produce the best outcomes at the least cost compared to other team members.

Unlike fee-for-service where the financial driver is providing services that generate the highest revenue, VBP is driven by who, what, where, and how services are provided that will achieve the healthcare goals of a patient or population and result in value, that is, a better health and healthcare experience at an acceptable cost. The premise is to develop and use the best care strategy and therapeutic plan possible in caring for a patient. Greater financial gain is realized when the organization can maximize the number of patients they serve, with efficient and wise use of team members. If CMM provided via telehealth is the optimal care strategy, that would be the course chosen without any question. Barriers and limitations such as professional territorialism and payment are no longer the pressures driving care decisions. The services provided are chosen based on those that are most cost-effective and meet patient needs in the most effective manner by the best qualified person. Using a provider who has medication management skills but who would be better utilized in diagnostic services or choosing a provider who may not have the knowledge to optimally and efficiently provide medication management does not make sense. VBP design creates an important opportunity for pharmacists, as they are the best healthcare team member to meet patient medication needs and improve medication-related health outcomes. Justification for services does not need to be based on revenue but rather on evidence of effectiveness. Experience and data gained from CMM provided via telehealth in the Veterans Affairs system and other systems suggest value through improving patient outcomes, satisfaction, access to care, and being a cost-effective option.[7-22]

FINANCIAL AND HEALTH IMPLICATIONS OF PHARMACY TELEHEALTH PRACTICES

While telehealth practices were growing prior to the public health emergency, the explosion of its use since the onset of the pandemic highlights the feasibility of its widespread use and brings up questions about impact on cost of care as well as health outcomes. There are no large-scale studies on the effects of telemedicine, nor is there consistency in defining what constitutes telemedicine. In 2016, the Agency for Healthcare Research and Quality (AHRQ) published a systematic review citing the effectiveness of both remote patient monitoring and counseling for patients with chronic conditions as well as behavioral health interventions. Similarly, interventions in blood glucose and hypertension management with remote monitoring and/or video-teleconferencing showed improvement in hemoglobin A1c and blood pressure in several studies.[23] A study utilizing a bedside assistant in a senior community to facilitate video telemedicine visits with primary care providers resulted in lower utilization of emergency departments.[24]

Overall, telemedicine shows promise to expand the reach of providers, improve chronic disease metrics, and reduce hospital and emergency department use. Further and more rigorous studies are needed to show the overall impact of pharmacy telehealth practice. Regulatory changes will prove to be an important factor in the ability to continue to scale these practices.

REFERENCES

1. CMS. National health expenditures 2019 highlights. **https://www.cms.gov/files/document/highlights.pdf**. Accessed May 13, 2021.
2. Tikkanen R, Abrams MK. U.S. Health Care from a Global Perspective, 2019: Higher Spending, Worse Outcomes? (Commonwealth Fund, January 2020). **https://doi.org/10.26099/7avy-fc29**. Accessed May 13, 2021.
3. Cutler DM. What is the US health spending problem? *Health Aff.* 2018;37:493-497.
4. Porter ME, Larsson S, Lee TH. Standardizing patient outcomes measurement. *N Engl J Med.* 2016;374:504-506.
5. Slone Epidemiology Center at Boston University. Patterns of Medication Use in the United States 2006. **https://www.bu.edu/slone/files/2012/11/SloneSurveyReport2006.pdf**. Accessed May 13, 2021.
6. Watanabe JH, McInnis T, Hirsch JD. Cost of prescription drug-related morbidity and mortality. *Ann Pharmacother.* 2018;52(9):829-837.
7. Singh LG, Accursi M, Korch-Black K. Implementation and outcomes of a pharmacist-managed clinical video telehealth anticoagulation clinic. *Am J Health Syst Pharm.* 2015;72(1):70-73.
8. Litke J, Spoutz, L, Ahlstrom D, et al. Impact of the clinical pharmacy specialist in telehealth primary care. *Am J Health-Syst Pharm.* 2018;75(13):982-986.
9. Margolis KL, Asche SE, Berdall AR, et al. Cardiovascular events and costs with home blood pressure telemonitoring and pharmacist management of uncontrolled HTN. *Hypertension* 2020;76:46-56.
10. Tetuan C, Axon DR, Bingham J, et al. Assessing the effect of a telepharmacist's recommendations during an integrated, interprofessional telehealth appointment and their alignment with quality measures. *J Manag Care Spec Pharm.* 2019;25(12):1334-1339.
11. Aberger EW, Migliozzi D, Follick MJ, et al. Enhancing patient engagement and blood pressure management for renal transplant recipients via home electronic monitoring and web-enabled collaborative care. *Telemed J E Health.* 2014;20(9):850-854.
12. Zullig LL, Jazowski SA, Davenport CA, et al. Primary care providers' acceptance of pharmacists' recommendations to support optimal medication management for patients with diabetic kidney disease. *J Gen Int Med.* 2019;35:63-69.
13. Leach M, Garcia G, Ganzer N. Implementation and evaluation of a pharmacist-run mental health treatment clinic via clinical video telehealth. *Ment Health Clin.* 2016;6(3):159-164.
14. Coakley C, Hough A, Dwyer D, Parra D. Clinical video telehealth in a cardiology pharmacotherapy clinic. *Am J Health Syst Pharm.* 2013 November 15;70(22):1974-1975.
15. Fortney JC, Pyne JM, Kimbrell TA, et al. Telemedicine-based collaborative care for posttraumatic stress disorder: A randomized clinical trial. *JAMA Psychiatry.* 2015;72(1):58-67.
16. Carter BL, Levy B, Gryzlak, B, et al. Cluster-randomized trial to evaluate a centralized clinical pharmacy service in private family medicine offices. *Circ Cardiovasc Qual Outcomes.* 018;11:e004188. doi: 10.1161/CIRCOUTCOMES.117.004188.
17. Dolder NM, Dolder CR. Comparison of a pharmacist managed lipid clinic: In-person versus telephone. *J Am Pharm Assoc.* 2010;50:375-378.
18. Crowley MJ, Edelman D, McAndrew AT, et al. Practical telemedicine for veterans with persistently poor diabetes control: A randomized pilot trial. *Telemedicine and E-Health.* 2016;22:376-384.
19. Zillich, Snyder ME, Frail CK, et al. A randomized, controlled pragmatic trial of telephonic medication therapy management to reduce hospitalization in home health patients. *Health Services Research.* 2014;49:1537-1554.
20. Magid, DJ, Ho PM, Olson KL, et al. A multi-modal blood pressure control intervention in 3 healthcare systems. *Am J Manag Care.* 2011;17(4):e96-e103.
21. Beran M, Asche SE, Bergdall AR, et al. Key components of success in a randomized trial of blood pressure telemonitoring with MTM pharmacists. *J Am Pharm Assoc.* 2018;58:614-621.
22. Ralston JD, Cook AJ, Anderson ML, et al. Home blood pressure monitoring, secure electronic messaging and medication intensification for improving HTN control. *Appl Clin Inf.* 2014;5:232-248.
23. Flodgren G, Rachas A, Farmer AJ, et al. Interactive telemedicine: Effects on professional practice and health care outcomes. *Cochrane Database System Rev.* 2015(9). Accessed May 13, 2021.
24. Shah, M, Wasserman E, Want H, et al. High-intensity telemedicine decreases emergency department use by senior living community residents. *Telemedicine and e-Health.* Mar 2016;251-258. Accessed May 13, 2021.

SECTION 3: CLINICAL VIGNETTE

Scenario 1

You are working through what billing opportunities might exist for your telehealth pharmacy services. You have considered using chronic care management (CCM) codes for your telehealth pharmacy services. As part of the workflow, you have established asynchronous data collection for important lab values (such as blood glucose monitoring) and vital signs (weight and blood pressure). Patients report their data through the electronic patient-facing portal of the electronic health record, so that you can review the information in advance of their telehealth pharmacy appointment. In your research, you came across remote physiologic monitoring (RPM) codes. Are RPM and CCM billable during the same month? With your workflow design of having patients submit data asynchronously via the patient-facing portal of the electronic health record, would you meet the criteria to bill RPM?

Response 1

RPM and CCM are billable during the same month. It is important to note that time spent on RPM cannot be counted toward the monthly CCM totals. In your workflow, you would need to ensure that your method for tracking time dedicated to CCM excludes time spent on RPM activities. When evaluating whether or not you can use RPM billing, it is critical to remember that the device used to collect patient data must upload data via digital means. Requirements also state that patient-reported data are not included in RPM billing. The workflow you have established does not include a device that allows for digital data upload, but is patient-reported data. This does not meet the requirements for RPM and would not be something you could implement with the workflow you have created.

Scenario 2

You have decided to pursue the use of chronic care management (CCM) billing codes for your telehealth pharmacy services. You have discussed it with clinic leadership and everyone agrees with pursuing CCM billing. Your clinic manager does ask to have a meeting with compliance to gain their approval before moving forward. This will be a new method of billing for the clinic, and the clinic manager wants to ensure that everything is in order before proceeding. In order to help the meeting run smoothly and be successful, what should you prepare ahead of time?

Response 2

To ensure a successful meeting with compliance, a great first step would be to outline all of the requirements for billing CCM. Once you have outlined all of the requirements, designate the specific pieces of the workflow that meet each of the requirements. For example, does your clinic have a 24/7 call service that can be used for patients receiving CCM? Is there a way to document patient consent electronically in a manner that provides automated prompts so that this step isn't missed? You will want to have each requirement outlined with a workflow step and with an explanation of how you will meet the requirement.

Often, pharmacists have to explain their scope and role to compliance officers. While the purpose of the meeting is not to discuss pharmacist scope and role, you may want to be prepared to do so. Providing documentation from state pharmacy practice acts that outline scope and cross-walking to how CCM fits within that scope can help facilitate a successful conversation with compliance.

SECTION 4
Tracking Metrics for Improved Care Quality, Increased Care Access, and Patient Experience

Eve M. Segal, Jeffery L. Olson, and Ashley Marie Parrott

CHAPTER 10
Understanding Quality Assessment Strategies and Applying Them to Telehealth Pharmacy Practice

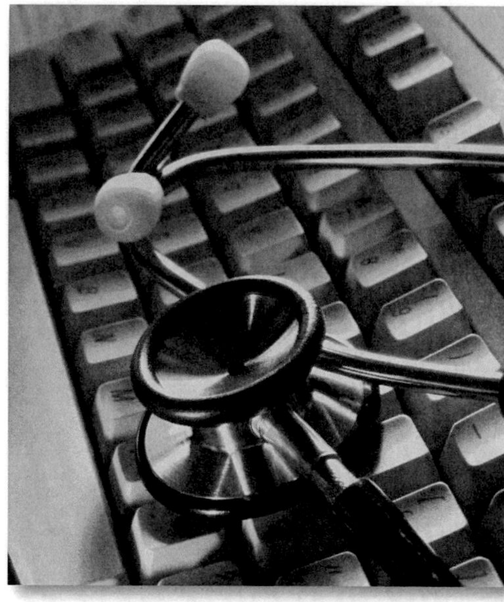

The framework for quality assurance (QA) has a long history in healthcare, stretching back centuries since the time of Hippocrates.[1] Medicine evolved into an evidence-based care culture, which is reflected in modern practice.[2] QA in healthcare is one of the top priorities for most providers and health organizations. This is because healthcare organizations recognize that QA programs can help prevent, detect, and potentially correct any problems that may arise in patients, which will translate into higher quality and standards of care.[3] Whereas QA is a structured and continuous program, quality assessment is the method for data collection and its subsequent analysis to which its results are compared to predefined standards.[4] QA programs have evolved significantly over time and are described below, from surveys evaluating hospital performance to establishing metrics for the digital age, like telehealth.

In the United States, an effort to achieve high-quality standards was developed gradually. Between 1995 and 2000, several quality improvement initiatives were performed.[5] Eventually, the Health Care Finance Administration (HCFA) identified quality indicators to routinely assess the excellence of care administered to its Medicare beneficiaries.[6] These quality indicators were broken into six domains of healthcare: safety, effectiveness, timeliness, patient-centeredness, efficiency, and equity.[7] The last three domains, as identified by the Institute of Medicine (IOM), are patient-centered and revolve around patient satisfaction or, in other words, patient experience. In general, quality indicators for healthcare are a vital tool used to track and evaluate the performance of an individual provider and a healthcare system. The specific indicators developed by HCFA focused on reviewing the impact of an intervention on the health status of a patient (e.g., percentage of patients diagnosed with hypertension with controlled blood pressures). Although this appeared to be the gold standard of assessing quality, relying solely on outcome measures to demonstrate therapeutic effectiveness has many drawbacks. Outcomes are the result of many contributing factors, many of which are out of an individual healthcare provider's control.

Parallel to the efforts of the HCFA, in 1994 the Healthcare Cost and Utilization Project (HCUP) created a set of quality indicators for hospitals, which was derived from discharge data. The Agency for Healthcare Research and Quality (AHRQ) maintains these commonly used indicators, which incorporate structural measures that address a provider's or a system's capacity (e.g., ratio of providers to patients) and process measures suggest what a provider does to improve health (e.g., percentage of patients who receive a preventive service like a screening colonoscopy).[8] Although AHRQ Quality Indicators (Qis) are used widely, many organizations have developed and use their own sets of quality indicators (**Table 10.1**). Most recently, some

DOI 10.37573/9781585286928.010

Table 10.1. AHRQ Quality Indicator Modules for Adult Patients[9]

Domain	Definition	Example Indicators
Prevention Quality Indicators (PQIs)	Calculates inpatient admissions that may have been avoided with access to outpatient care.	• Diabetes short-term complication admission rate • Perforated appendix admission rate • Diabetes long-term complication admission rate • Chronic obstructive pulmonary disease admission rate • Hypertension admission rate • Congestive heart failure (CHF) admission rate • Low birth weight rate • Dehydration admission rate • Bacterial pneumonia admission rate • Urinary tract infection admission rate • Angina admission without procedure • Uncontrolled diabetes admission rate • Adult asthma admission rate • Rate of lower-extremity amputation among patients with diabetes
Inpatient Quality Indicators (IQIs): Provider-Level Volume	Focuses on volume and measures the total amount of admissions and procedures performed.	• Esophageal resection volume • Pancreatic resection volume • Abdominal aortic aneurysm (AAA) repair volume • Coronary artery bypass graft (CABG) volume • Percutaneous transluminal coronary angioplasty (PTCA) volume • Carotid endarterectomy (CEA) volume
IQIs: Mortality Indicators	Includes indicators that cover procedures where higher mortality is associated with poorer care.	• Esophageal resection mortality rate • Pancreatic resection mortality rate • AAA repair mortality rate • CABG mortality rate • PTCA mortality rate • CEA mortality rate • Craniotomy mortality rate • Hip replacement mortality rate
IQIs: Mortality Indicators with Varying Mortality Rates	Describes procedures where volumes vary throughout the country. These indicators cover procedures where higher mortality rate is associated with poorer care.	• Acute myocardial infarction (AMI) mortality rate • AMI mortality rate, without transfer cases • CHF mortality rate • Acute stroke morality rate • Gastrointestinal hemorrhage mortality rate • Hip fracture mortality rate • Pneumonia mortality rate
IQIs: Utilization Indicators	Includes indicators that measure high or low rates of specific procedures. High or low rates for these indicators represent inappropriate care delivery.	• Cesarean section delivery rate • Primary cesarean delivery rate • Vaginal birth after cesarean (VBAC) rate • VBAC rate, uncomplicated • Laparoscopic cholecystectomy rate • Incidental appendectomy in the elderly rate • Bilateral cardiac catherization rate

Domain	Definition	Example Indicators
Patient Safety Indicators (PSIs): Provider-level	Uses hospital inpatient discharge data to understand patient safety. Focuses on postoperative complications, adverse events, challenges with procedures, and trauma related to birth.	• Postoperative pulmonary embolism or deep vein thrombosis • Postoperative respiratory failure • Postoperative sepsis • Postoperative physiologic and/or metabolic derangements • Postoperative abdominopelvic wound dehiscence • Postoperative hip fracture • Postoperative hemorrhage or hematoma • Decubitus ulcer • Selected infections due to medical care • Iatrogenic pneumothorax • Accidental puncture or laceration • Foreign body left in during procedure • Birth trauma resulting in injury to neonate • Obstetric trauma due to vaginal delivery with instrument • Obstetric trauma from a vaginal delivery without an instrument • Obstetric trauma related to cesarean section delivery • Complication of anesthesia • Death in low-mortality diagnosis-related groups (DRGs) • Death in surgical inpatients with treatable serious complications (a previously known failure to rescue) • Transfusion reactions (AB/Rh)

organizations have been developing quality indicators for telehealth, which will be described later in this chapter.

After these quality indicators were developed, public reporting efforts began in 2006 under the Physician Quality Reporting Initiative (PQRI). Under the Tax Relief and Health Care Act (TRHCA) of 2006, PQRI enacted a pay-for-reporting system. This program focused on providing a formal mechanism for healthcare providers to evaluate and improve the quality of the care they provide to Medicare beneficiaries.[10] The program provided incentive payments, which consisted of a 1.5% bond on Medicare Part B fee-for-service (FFS) charges for successful reporting on three quality measures. Then, in 2008, the Medicare Improvement for Patients and Providers Act (MIPPA) was enacted, and the incentive payments were increased to 2%.[5] Although this was the beginning of formalized quality assurance programs, the Patient Protection and Accountable Care Act which was signed into law in 2010 highlighted the importance of a continuous quality program in healthcare.[5] The overarching goal of this law was to improve quality of care, expand access, and lower healthcare costs for Medicare and Medicaid beneficiaries. To achieve this goal, the Patient-Centered Outcomes Research Institute (PCORI) was launched and began researching the effectiveness of various clinical interventions determining which treatments were the most effective for various patient populations. These findings guided evidence-based treatment algorithms to ensure high-quality care is maintained. In 2015, the Medicare Access and CHIP Reauthorization Act (MACRA) was passed. This law transitioned payments to the Merit-based Incentive Payment System (MIPS), which incorporates alternative payment models and merit-based payment systems.[11] MIPS combines three of CMS's value-based programs: the physician quality reporting system, the value-based payment modifier, and the Medicare electronic health record (EHR) incentive program.[12] Although this value-base model can be utilized across inpatient and outpatient facilities, because of this combination of reporting programs many outpatient providers and organizations have elected to enroll in MIPS payment models. Overall, 280 quality measures have been identified (**Table 10.2**).[11]

Table 10.2. Example of MIPS Quality Measures[13]

Heart failure (HF): beta-blocker therapy for left ventricular systolic dysfunction (LVSD)
Urinary Incontinence: assessment of presence or absence of urinary incontinence in women aged 65 or older
Urinary incontinence: plan of care for urinary incontinence in women aged 65 years or older
Chronic obstructive pulmonary disease (COPD): long-acting inhaled bronchodilator therapy
Prostate cancer: avoidance of overuse of bone scan for staging low-risk prostate cancer patients
Prostate cancer: combination androgen deprivation therapy for high-risk or very high-risk prostate cancer
Preventive care screening: body mass index (BMI) screening and follow-up plan

TELEHEALTH AND QUALITY ASSURANCE STRATEGIES

Telehealth encounters have surged during the COVID-19 pandemic. In a study by Koonin and colleagues, telehealth visits increased substantially from 2019 through 2020. For example, in the first quarter of 2020, there was a 50% increase in telehealth visits compared to the same period in 2019.[14] In another report by the Mayo Clinic, in-person visits declined a dramatic 78% during the COVID-19 pandemic from mid-March to mid-April. However, during that same time, telehealth was widely utilized, and the health system reported an astonishing 10,880% increase in this digital healthcare service.[15] Although there has been a large effort to develop quality measures for in-person visits in inpatient and outpatient settings, these assessments for telehealth are lacking. Patients have generally responded positively to telehealth as a means of obtaining healthcare. Studies have demonstrated that patients are generally satisfied with telehealth services and report that saving time is a primary benefit of digital platforms.[16,17] However, for all the purported benefits that telehealth has provided for patients and healthcare providers, the need to ensure that patients are deriving the same benefit from a digital health visit that they would receive from an in-person visit remains. Prior to the COVID-19 pandemic, several studies questioned if a telehealth platform is a more advantageous way to measure, track, and report the quality of care given to patients.[18] But with the widespread adoption of telehealth as a means of managing acute and chronic health conditions, the question of quality assessment for this visit type remains even more paramount.

Patient Experience

Patient experience is often tied to essential quality indicators. However, measuring the patient experience has been challenging. In 2008, with passage of MIPPA there was also a provision to assess the patient experience as part of the quality assessment. A variety of surveys have been used to measure patient encounters in both hospitals and outpatient clinics, but MIPPA tied these metrics to financial reimbursements, as detailed above.[5,19] A variety of surveys have been used in the ambulatory setting such as the Consumer Assessment of Healthcare Providers and Systems Clinician and Group (CG-CAHPS) survey for outpatient surgery and the National Ambulator Medical Care Survey (NAMCS), or the Ambulatory Care Experiences Survey (ACES). Press Ganey's CG-CAHPS is one of the most widely used and validated patient experience surveys. It assesses the patient experience of adults and children in ambulatory or specialized care (**Table 10.3**). By weaving in the patient perspective with these quality indicators, the approach to quality becomes more holistic and allows care to be patient-centered and embody a team-based approach. Efforts like this provide national benchmarks for patient outcomes in a structured manner that assists healthcare professionals and organizations to provide high-quality evidence-based care to their patients.

Table 10.3. Select Quality Indicators for Telehealth: NQF Recommendations[28]

Domain	Subdomain	Measure Concept
Experience	Patient, family, and/or caregiver	Overall improvement in quality of life because services are received at home
Experience	Patient, family, and/or caregiver	Patients able to interpret diagnosis and treatment instructions through telehealth
Experience	Patient, family, and/or caregiver	Decrease in wait times for patients
Financial impact/cost	Financial impact on health system or payer	Visit duration measured versus in-home care
Financial impact/cost	Financial impact on care team	Decrease in no-show rate
Access to care	Access for care team	In-person visit agreed to after a telehealth consultation
Access to care	Access for care team and for patient, family, and/or caregiver	Number of interprofessional visits
Effectiveness	System effectiveness	Amount of time to schedule a visit
Effectiveness	System effectiveness	Amount of time to check in for a visit
Effectiveness	Clinical effectiveness	Relationship of the telehealth modality to the therapeutic need of the patient
Effectiveness	Operational effectiveness	Can telehealth offer similar quality of services across a population of similar patients?

Example of CG-CAHPS Survey Questions[20]

Each using the scale: [1]☐Very poor [2]☐Poor [3]☐Fair [4]☐Good [5]☐Very good

- Friendliness/courtesy of the care providers
- Explanations the care provider gave you about your problem or condition
- Concern the care provider showed for your questions or worries
- Care provider's efforts to include you in decisions about your treatment
- Information the care provider gave you about medications (if any)
- Instructions the care provider gave you about follow-up care (if any)
- Degree to which the care provider talked with you using words you could understand
- Amount of time the care provider spent with you
- Your confidence in this care provider
- Likelihood of your recommending this care provider to others

Telehealth Pharmacy Practice Patient Experience

Assessing the patient experience with telehealth across different demographics and socioeconomic situations is essential for organizations. In general, patients appear to be very satisfied with the telehealth platform to access their healthcare providers. In a retrospective single-center cohort study in New York City, 38,609 Press Ganey patient satisfaction surveys were evaluated and found that scores were significantly higher (94.9% vs. 92.5%; $p < 0.001$) compared to in-person visits.[21] Compared to in-person visits, there are several ways beyond the survey to assess patient experience with telehealth. For example, other key data points can be passively pulled which illuminate a patient's preferences to the telehealth platform. For example, identifying patient visits as either telephone only, video only, or in-person can help determine patient preferences. Organizations can also use custom patient survey questions to glean information on telehealth quality and the patient experience. By asking questions regarding time or money saved, access to technology and preference of using this technology can help organizations understand the patient experience with telehealth. An alternative to developing internal patient survey questions is to use established questionnaires to measure the patient experience. Commonly used validated surveys include the Telehealth Usability Questionnaire (TUQ) or the Telemedicine Satisfaction and Usefulness Questionnaire.[22] These questionnaires assess usefulness, ease of use, quality of the telehealth interface, quality of the interaction with telehealth, reliability of the system, and patient experience.[23,24]

Clinical Quality Audits

With this infrastructure, benchmark reporting, and methodology being set at a national level, it is critical that individual provider groups and organizations understand how to perform a clinical quality audit. The clinical audit is a key part of the quality improvement process, but it is also a measure of effectiveness. In general, it requires measuring the outcomes achieved against established standards, which were reviewed above. It is crucial to understand that the clinical audit goes beyond data collection. Successful clinical audits measure patient outcomes against standards or defined quality indicators, with the expectation of improving that practice. Clinical audits should be repeated frequently to ensure that any changes made to a practice demonstrate improvement.[25] The first step to a successful clinical audit is to identify the topic to be evaluated. The ideal topic should be one that meets the following benchmarks:[25]

- High volume of work
- Risky
- Highly variable
- Complex
- Potentially innovative

An overview of how to perform a clinical audit is drawn in **Figure 10.1**. Following proper identification of a topic, the scope of the project should be developed along with the corresponding methodology. The goal of the audit could be to evaluate a new process (e.g., patient adherence to warfarin using a telehealth platform) and/or improvement of a current process.[26] Once the topic is identified and its corresponding methodology is developed, quality indicators should be selected. With these two key pieces of information defined, data collection can begin. This data collection may be performed either prospectively or retrospectively. The data itself can be quantitative or qualitative and include elements such as surveys, interviews, and questionnaires.[27] Discrete data points from medical records like lab results or diagnosis codes can be included. A patient's medical record is primarily the main source of information for most clinical audits, but it is important to know that it may be lacking all the required data points needed.[25] Following data collection, a comparison of your collected data with the benchmark standards must occur. This is the cornerstone of the clinical audit. Results from this comparison can demonstrate whether a standard is met and ultimately that further improvement is needed. If results are close to the standard used, then the clinical audit can enter a monitoring phase.[25,27] Lastly, the cycle ends with change implementation. Following a change, it is important to go back and perform the clinical audit again to ensure that the changes made were positive and align with the standards previously identified.[27]

Telehealth Clinical Quality Audits

Identifying clinical outcome targets is as important as identifying quality outcomes. Although this is currently ill defined and the overall data are lacking, the rapid adoption of telehealth offers an opportunity to compare outcome measures following telehealth and in-person visits among patients with chronic health conditions like heart disease and diabetes. Although telehealth may

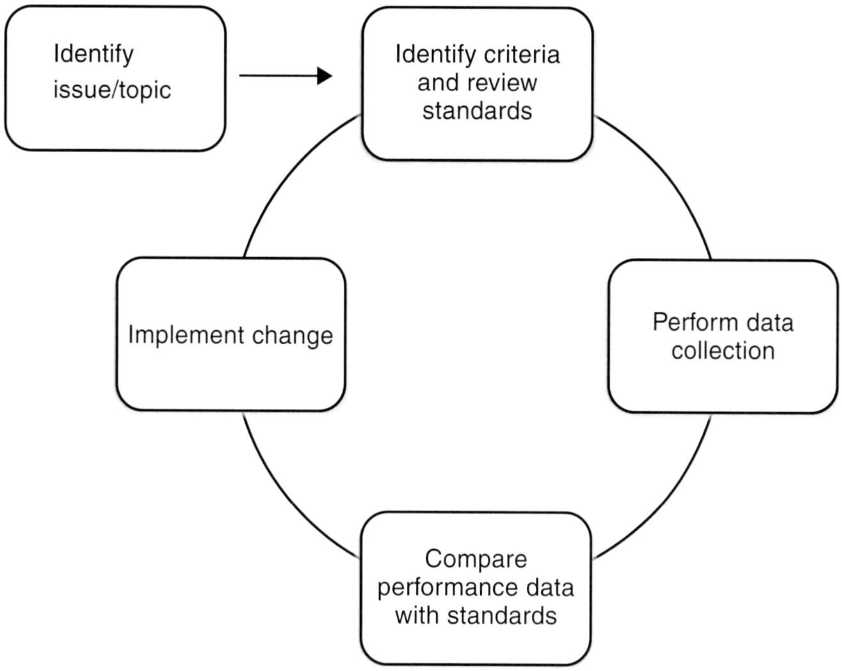

FIGURE 10.1. Key Components of the clinical audit process. Adapted from Ashmore S, Ruthven T. Clinical audit: a guide. *Nursing Management (Harrow)*, 2008;15(1):18-22.

offer opportunities to increase patient compliance, pharmacists must follow recommended and evidence-based practices when they provide care through this modality.

To perform clinical audits of telehealth, it is important that key indicators be abstracted in a chart review (Table 10.3). Having components like a telehealth consent and indicators about mode of technology used for a patient visit can make this abstraction easier. Lastly, it is crucial that organizations evaluate medication safety within the telehealth context. Reviewing charts for adverse events and creating voluntary reporting tools to catch medication errors related to telehealth are essential.

When you are determining which metrics to track for a telehealth service, it may be worthwhile to evaluate any metrics that are being tracked for a similar in-person service. Often, the goals of a service may be very similar regardless of whether the service is being delivered in person or by using telehealth. To date, very little has been published on the effectiveness of pharmacy services provided via traditional methods (i.e., face to face) compared with telehealth services.

Medication Safety

Routine clinical quality audits are one piece of the quality assurance puzzle. A key component of quality assurance for any organization is ensuring safe practices for patients. One way to improve practice is through a medication safety review. Medication errors and medication-related adverse events have serious ramifications in patient care. Errors due to healthcare are the fourth leading cause of death in the United States and the leading cause of preventable death.[29] Medication errors are also associated with increased length of hospital stays and additional costs. Therefore, to prevent erroneous morbidity and mortality from medication-related adverse events or errors, detection of these events is a paramount step.

Table 10.4. Commonly Used Methods to Assess Medication Errors and Adverse Events[30]

Method	Advantages	Disadvantages	Efficacy
Chart abstraction/ review	• Retroactive • Uses standardized criteria	• Time consuming • Labor-intensive	Gold standard to detect adverse events
Claims data	• Uses local data • Captures unapparent failures	• Litigation based and may have legal implications	Adverse events detected
Incident reporting (sentinel events)	• High-quality data • Captures active and unapparent failures	• Only identifies severe, unexplained events or deaths • Can underestimate rates of adverse events • May cause feelings of blame, fear of punishment	• Contributes to reports and alerting • Measures adverse events
Voluntary reporting	• Variety of sources can report events • Uses a structured and simplified form • Captures active and unapparent failures • Promotes a culture of safety	• Variable quality of reporting • Underreporting • Individuals may feel the tool contributes to a blame culture • No data integration	• Contributes to reports and alerting • Provides path for feedback and opportunities for corrective actions • Medication errors are detected
Computer monitoring	• Multidata source integration • Real time • Adverse event prevention	• Poor software • Poor triggers • Undetermined future risks • Inadvertent errors in data inserted	• Captures prescribing faults • Captures prescription errors • Captures dispensing errors
Direct care observation	• Accurate • Captures active errors	• Time consuming • Difficult to train	• Data are centralized around administration errors
Patient monitoring	• Data from outpatients • Wide impacts	• Tools are not standardized and vary (interviews, questionnaires, focus groups, etc.)	• Can help direct future developments of patient-centered care

On a national level, various regulatory agencies and federal organizations collect data and create standardized recommendations or alerts, such as the Food and Drug Administration MedWatch program, the Joint Commission on the Accreditation of Healthcare Organizations, and the Institute of Safe Medication Practices. However, individual organizations must also develop tools to analyze errors and identify areas to improve quality and make system changes. In order to monitor safe medication processes, organizations must evaluate both adverse events and medication errors. However, the methods used to evaluate each of these categories varies. Most organizations use chart review to detect adverse events. By utilizing monitoring tools within the electronic health record, incident reporting, or auditing claims data, adverse events can be passively pulled and demonstrate clinical outcomes for the entire patient population in question.[30] Medication errors are primarily detected by direct observation and voluntary reporting. Most organizations have employee reporting tools such as the Patient Safety Net (PSN) through which healthcare providers can summarize a patient event and each event undergoes a root cause analysis. Detection methods commonly used to assess medication errors are outlined in **Table 10.4**. Organizations can use these events to implement changes. Interestingly, the adoption of telemedicine may result in a reduction of medication and medical errors. A study using remote pharmacist review of medication orders for three community hospitals found an increase in interventions resulting in improved patient safety.[31] By leveraging this technology, patient safety can be optimized in new ways; however, more data are needed to support patient safety benefits.

Maintaining Quality and Safety with Pharmacy Telehealth Practice

At the time of this writing, standardized quality assessment and assurance approaches to telehealth pharmacy practice models have largely not been developed. In fact, national conversations about this topic are ongoing. However, thanks to the above-outlined robust quality initiatives that have taken place over the past three decades, we can incorporate existing approaches and modify them to a telehealth pharmacy practice visit. To perform a quality assessment, it is imperative that quality indicators be identified. Nonprofits like the National Quality Forum (NQF) are attempting to develop standardized quality indicators for telehealth that focus on access to care, financial impacts or cost, the telehealth experience, and effectiveness of treatment. However, benchmarks are currently not well defined and need to be further developed.

REFERENCES

1. De Jonge V, Sint Nicolaas J, van Leerdam M, et al. Overview of the quality assurance movement in health care. *Best Pract Res Clin Gastroenterol*. 2011;25(3):337-347. doi: 10.1016/j.bpg.2011.05.001.
2. Guyatt G, Cook D, Haynes B. Evidence based medicine has come a long way. *BMJ*. 2004;329(7473): 990-991. doi: 10.1136/bmj.329.7473.990.
3. Institute of Medicine (US) Committee to Design a Strategy for Quality Review and Assurance in Medicare; Lohr KN (ed). *Medicare: A Strategy for Quality Assurance*: Volume 1. Washington, DC: National Academies Press, 1990. 9, Methods of Quality Assessment and Assurance. **https://www.ncbi.nlm.nih.gov/books/NBK235459**.
4. Mainz J, Hammershøy EM, Worning AM, et al. Quality assessment, quality assurance and quality improvement in health care. Concepts and terminology. *Ugeskr Laeger*. 1992;154(17):1151-1156.
5. Marjoua Y, Bozic K. Brief history of quality movement in US healthcare. *Curr Rev Musculoskelet Med*. 2012;5(4):265-273. doi: 10.1007/s12178-012-9137-8.
6. Jencks SF, Cuerdon T, Burwen DR, et al. Quality of medical care delivered to Medicare beneficiaries: A profile at state and national levels. *JAMA*. 2000;284:1670-1676. doi: 10.1001/jama.284.13.1670.
7. Berwick DM. A user's manual for the IOM's "Quality Chasm" Report. *Health Aff*. 2002;21(3):80-90. doi: 10.1377/hlthaff.21.3.80.
8. Types of health care quality measures. (n.d.). **https://www.ahrq.gov/talkingquality/measures/types.html**. Accessed on May 18, 2021.
9. Farquhar M. AHRQ Quality indicators. In: Hughes RG (ed). *Patient Safety and Quality: An Evidence-Based Handbook for Nurses*. Rockville, MD: Agency for Healthcare Research and Quality; 2008 Apr. Chapter 45. **https://www.ncbi.nlm.nih.gov/books/NBK2664**. Accessed May 18, 2021.
10. Dowd B, Li CH, Swenson T, et al. Medicare's Physician Quality Reporting System (PQRS): Quality measurement and beneficiary attribution. *Medicare Medicaid Res Rev*. 2014 Jun 25;4(2). doi: 10.5600/mmrr.004.02.a04.
11. Manchikanti L, Hammer M, Benyamin R, et al. Merit-based incentive payment system (MIPS): Harsh choices for interventional pain management physicians. *Pain Physician*. 2016;19:E15-E32.
12. Yon K, Sinclair J, Bentley OS, et al. Impact of quality measures performed through pharmacist collaboration with a primary care clinic. *J Am Pharm Assoc*. 2003; 2020;60(3 S): S97-S102. **https://doi.org/10.1016/j.japh.2020.01.011**.
13. 2020 Annual Call for Quality Measures Fact Sheet. (2020, May 22). Retrieved May 06, 2021. **https://www.cms.gov/files/document/2020-mips-call-quality-measure-overview-fact-sheet.pdf**
14. Koonin L, Hoots B, Tsang C, et al. Trends in the use of telehealth during the emergence of the COVID-19 pandemic—United States, January-March 2020. *Weekly*. 2020;69(43):1595-1599.
15. Demaerschalk B, Blegen R, Ommen S. Scalability of telemedicine services in a large integrated multispecialty health care system during COVID-19. *Telemed e-Health*. 2021:96-98. **http://doi.org/10.1089/tmj.2020.0290**.
16. Polinski JM, Barker T, Gagliano N, et al. Patients' satisfaction with and preference for telehealth visits. *J Gen Intern Med*. 2016 Mar;31(3):269-275. doi: 10.1007/s11606-015-3489-x.
17. Jacobs J, Ferguson J, Van Campen J, et al. Organizational and external factors associated with video telehealth use in the veterans' health administration before and during the COVID-19 pandemic. *Telemedicine and e-Health*. 2021. doi: **http://doi.org/10.1089/tmj.2020.0530**.
18. Halpren-Ruder D, Chang A, Hollander J, et al. Quality assurance in telehealth: Adherence to evidence-based indicators. *Telemed J E Health*. 2019;25(7):599-603. doi: 10.1089/tmj.2018.0149.
19. Mazurenko O, Collum T, Ferdinand A, et al. Predictors of hospital patient satisfaction as measured by HCAHPS. *J Healthcare Manag*. 2017;62(4):272-283. doi: 10.1097/JHM-D-15-00050.
20. An overview of Version 3.0 of the CAHPS Clinician & Group Survey. (2015, June 17). Retrieved May 6, 2021. **https://www.ahrq.gov/sites/default/files/wysiwyg/cahps/surveys-guidance/cg/about/cg_3-0_overview.pdf**.
21. Ramaswamy A, Yu M, Drrangsholt S, et al. Patient satisfaction with telemedicine during the COVID-19 pandemic: Retrospective cohort study. *J Med Internet Res* 2020;22(9):e20786. doi: 10.2196/20786.
22. Chuo J, Macy ML, Lorch SA. Strategies for evaluating telehealth. *Pediatrics* 2020 Nov;146(5):e20201781. doi: 10.1542/peds.2020-1781.

23. Parmanto B, Lewis Jr A, Graham K, et al. Development of the telehealth usability questionnaire (TUQ). *Int J Telerehabil*. 2016;8(1);3-10. doi: 10.5195/ijt.2016.6196.

24. Bakken S, Grullon-Figueroa L, Izquierdo R, et al. Development, validation, and use of English and Spanish versions of the telemedicine satisfaction and usefulness questionnaire. *J Am Med Inform Assoc*. 2006l 13(6):660-667. doi: 10.1197/jamia.M2146.

25. Esposito P, Dal Canton A. Clinical audit, a valuable tool to improve quality of care: General methodology and applications in nephrology. *World J Nephrol*. 2014;3(4):249-255. doi: 10.5527/wjn.v3.i4.249.

26. Buth S, D'Cruz L. Clinical audit—process and outcome for improved clinical practice. *Dent Update*. 2012;39:710-714. doi: 10.12968/denu.2012.39.10.710.

27. Soimakallio S, Alanen A, Jarvinen H, et al. Clinical audit: Development of the criteria of good practices. *Radiat Prot Dosimetry*. 2011;147(1-2):30-33. doi: 10.1093/rpd/ncr260.

28. Creating a framework to support measure development for telehealth. (2017, August). **http://www.qualityforum.org/Publications/2017/08/Creating_a_Framework_to_Support_Measure_Development_for_Telehealth.aspx**. Accessed May 18, 2021.

29. Light D, Lexchin J, Darrow J. Institutional corruption of pharmaceuticals and the myth of safe and effective drugs. *J Law, Med Ethics*. 2013;14(3):590-610. doi: 10.1111/jlme.12068.

30. Montesi G, Lechi A. Prevention of medication errors: Detection and audit. *Br J Clin Pharmacol*. 2009;67(6):651-655. doi: 10.1111/j.1365-2125.2009.03422.x.

31. Schneider PJ. Evaluating the impact of telepharmacy. *Am J Health Syst Pharm*. 2013;70:2130-2135. doi: 10.2146/ajhp130138.

CHAPTER 11
Identifying Types of Metrics for Telehealth Evaluation

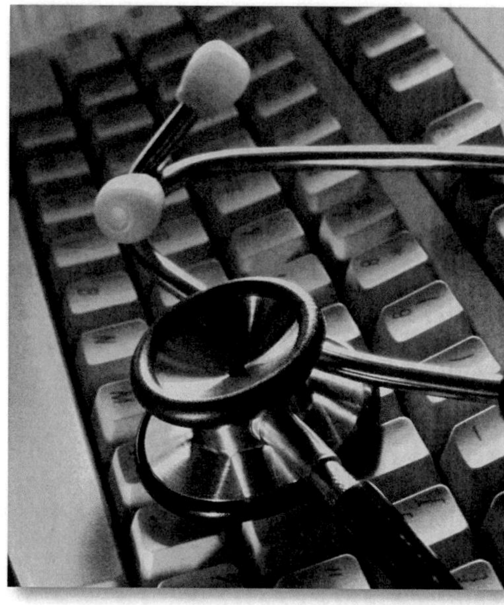

Metrics serve a valuable purpose across business and healthcare settings. Identifying the correct metrics can lead to improved patient care, profitability, and success. Selecting the wrong metric can lead to patient dissatisfaction, employee discouragement, financial losses, and potentially even failure. By establishing key performance indicators (KPIs), one is able to focus work on the most important and meaningful metrics. If set properly, KPIs will provide valuable focus to leaders and front-line employees. A thoughtful approach to metric selection is an essential aspect of developing successful telehealth services.

Metrics can be broken down and organized in multiple ways. Each individual organization likely has their preferred method, which is often aligned to the mission, vision, and values of the organization. Understanding your organization's priorities will prove valuable in determining the best way to organize metrics for a telehealth service. Further, that understanding will help you prioritize which metrics to focus efforts around. Of equal importance, organizational priorities will help you determine which metrics are less important.

Many of the metrics used to assess telehealth services do not vary significantly from traditional metrics that you might choose to evaluate a service delivered by more traditional means. This can be helpful while establishing telehealth services because previously established metrics can be immediately employed in tracking and assessing services delivered remotely. Adjustments and metric additions will further enhance effective measurement of telehealth services. The discussion surrounding different types of metrics will include those you might find with ambulatory care services delivered face-to-face that can be applied to care delivered virtually, along with metrics that might be considered more exclusive to telehealth services.

In this chapter we divide metrics into five general categories: access to care, financial impact/cost, experience, effectiveness, and utilization. This breakdown aligns with the domains that the National Quality Forum (NQF) outlined in its telehealth report published in 2017 (which was introduced in Table 10.3). The classification of metrics was based on a comprehensive environmental scan of available publications surrounding telehealth measures.

Tool for telehealth pharmacy practice evaluation: Utilizing a framework to select, organize, and communicate key performance indicators will position one well for demonstrating value and justifying service expansion. Aligning metrics with organizational priorities and goals is important. Remember that continual improvement and refinement of metric tracking will be needed.

DOI 10.37573/9781585286928.011

Table 11.1. Examples and Definitions of Access Metrics

Access Metric Examples	Definition
Median lag time	Number of days to the next available appointment
Third next available	Average length of time in days between the request for an appointment and the third available appointment
Future capacity	Percent of time available to book patients for the next 4 weeks
Panel size	Number of unique patients attributed to an individual provider

FIVE CATEGORIES OF METRICS

Access to Care

The access to care domain focuses on whether remote individuals can obtain needed information, expertise, or clinical services effectively. A significant driver behind implementing telehealth services is to improve patient access to care. It also includes connecting clinical experts to healthcare professionals in areas where those experts may be lacking.

As stated previously, meaningful access metrics will vary depending on your ambulatory practice, the services or information being delivered, and the priorities of the organization or practice. A few examples are provided in **Table 11.1**.

Financial Impact

The financial impact domain includes measures that assess revenues, expenses, and cost savings attributed to delivery of a service. The ultimate decision as to whether a telehealth pharmacy practice service is implemented comes down to its financial viability. Clearly defined, accurate financial metrics can create a strong case for implementation or continued support of a service.

The financial impact of the delivery of care is of great concern to various individuals and groups. Patients, families, and/or caregivers value reduced out-of-pocket expense. Demonstrating reduced costs to patients through telehealth services is a valuable selling point. Telehealth services that deliver reduced out-of-pocket savings, while still delivering quality care, are attractive for patients. Members of the care team also celebrate opportunities to reduce a patient's costs.

Health systems value reduced overhead and operational costs. Depending on a health system's priorities, different metrics might be more meaningful. For example, per member per month (PMPM) savings would be meaningful to an organization operating in a value-based environment, where profit per encounter or relative value unit (RVU) might be more appropriate in a health system with more emphasis on fee-for-service.

Payers are drawn to measures that demonstrate reduced overall cost. PMPM savings (medical and pharmaceutical) are one example. Generic prescribing and formulary compliance percentages can also demonstrate value to payers. Examples and definitions of other metrics related to financials and cost are presented in **Table 11.2**.

Experience

The experience domain centers on the usability and participation in a telehealth pharmacy practice encounter. The focus on the consumer or patient experience is growing within healthcare. With more healthcare information from both credible and suspect sources easily accessible to patients, providing a valuable patient experience will help draw patients to quality care delivered by clinical professionals.

Table 11.2. Examples and Definitions of Metrics Related to Financials and Cost of Care

Financial Impact/Cost Metric Examples	Definition
Out-of-pocket cost savings	Patient costs for healthcare services or products received. Does not include insurance premiums.
Per member per month (PMPM)	Metric used by payers to describe the average cost of healthcare for each member
Profit or savings per encounter	Financial savings/profit per unit allows for scaling of services
% formulary compliance	Ratio of alignment with a payer's formulary. Increased compliance leads to pharmaceutical expense savings
% generic prescribing	Ratio of generic medications prescribed compared to overall prescribing
Return on investment (ROI)	The financial return on an investment made or expenses realized
Relative value unit (RVU)	Measurement of provider productivity

Table 11.3. Examples and Definitions of Experience Metrics

Experience Metric Examples	Definition
Net promotor score	Metric that shows a customer's overall satisfaction of a service
Likelihood to recommend	An example of a customer service question that describes a customer's likelihood to recommend your service
Provider satisfaction	Similar to customer satisfaction, measuring providers' satisfaction for services provided by ambulatory care pharmacists via telehealth adds value to providers and their patients
Well-being index	Measure of healthcare professional burnout. With levels of burnout increasing, it is valuable to measure and share services that can improve the well-being of pharmacists and physicians.
Customer service stories	Stories that describe the care delivered connect to an individual's emotions and can describe the individual impact that makes numbers and percentages more personal.

Customer service is valued across service industries. It is tied to consumer satisfaction and loyalty. The patient's experience also plays a role in the perceived quality of care. Metrics evaluating patient experience might include net promotor score or likelihood to recommend. Tracking and sharing stories of excellent customer service are also important.

Employee and provider experience are also valuable to measure. Happy and satisfied employees tend to lead to better patient care and better patient experience. For pharmacists delivering care to patients in ambulatory care settings, provider satisfaction can be a significant driver for both the care team and the broader health system. Examples of experience metrics can be found in **Table 11.3**.

Effectiveness

The effectiveness domain encompasses a large variety of potentially important metrics for an ambulatory care pharmacy service. Quality measures and metrics are a core part of the effectiveness domain. System, clinical, operational, and technical effectiveness measures are meaningful. Examples and definitions of effectiveness metrics can be found in **Table 11.4**.

Table 11.4. Examples and Definitions of Effectiveness Metrics

Effectiveness Metric Examples	Definition
Population health targets	Numerous priority population health targets could be identified and used.
Disease markers	Blood pressure, HbA1c, INR, cholesterol, etc.
Time to goal	More rapid achievement of therapy goals demonstrates the effectiveness of pharmacist and telehealth services.
Readmission rates	Reductions in costly readmission rates demonstrate impactful cost savings and improved quality of care.
Event occurrence rates	Reductions in complications or events demonstrate the effectiveness of services.
Medication therapy problems identified/resolved	Identification and resolution of medication therapy problems highlight the impact pharmacists have in improving patient safety and care quality.
Telehealth cases	Both telehealth encounters and ratios of telehealth encounters to overall patient encounters can be meaningful to detail the work being done.

Table 11.5. Examples and Definitions of Utilization Metrics

Utilization Metric	Definition
Percentage of population engaged in initial visit	Number of unique patients engaged in an initial visit/total population eligible for service
Percentage of population engaged in follow-up visits	Number of unique patients engaged in a second visit (follow-up visit)/number of unique patients engaged in an initial visit

System metrics might include effective sharing of information between different healthcare professionals and population health targets (i.e., medication adherence, health screening completion). Clinical metrics include both direct and indirect outcome and process measures of quality. Disease markers (HbA1c, blood pressure, etc.), readmission rates, event occurrence, and medication therapy problems are only some metrics that may be valuable to track.

Operational effectiveness might include metrics that demonstrate integration into the broader health system. Being able to speak **to** the volume and types of services delivered by various telehealth means (i.e., synchronous, asynchronous, remote patient monitoring, mobile health applications) can demonstrate operational effectiveness.

As with other telehealth domains, selection of metrics will depend greatly on individual practice and health-system priorities. Careful selection of the highest priority metrics can increase visibility and demonstrate value to multiple stakeholders.

Utilization

While the utilization of a service is not defined in the NQF telehealth report, it is an important consideration that is often overlooked. For those services that require a provider referral to the pharmacist, the number of referrals compared to the number of eligible patients should be measured. For any type of pharmacist service, evaluating how frequently patients are engaging in the service is also important. Evaluating the number of unique patient referrals compared to the number of unique patient initial visits can provide a snapshot of how well your patient engagement strategies are working (**Table 11.5**). Comparing the type of visit in which patients engage can also provide some insight into the uptake of in-person visits versus telehealth visits, helping to tailor the service to fit the needs of the population.

Countless metrics exist across the domains of access to care, financial impacts, experience, effectiveness, and utilization. A common misstep is to track "everything." While this approach seems reasonable, especially if data are readily available, it can dilute and even hide the most meaningful measures. Selecting KPIs will allow you and stakeholders to focus on the most important and most impactful metrics. Demonstrating value and continuous improvement across a few metrics is often preferable to measuring everything. Selecting metrics that align with organizational priorities and reimbursement strategies may help you to be the most successful.

This chapter provides a framework for understanding and organizing different types of metrics available for helping to communicate a powerful story about the work being delivered via telehealth. Understanding different types of metrics and prioritizing the most impactful will position you well to communicate meaningfully to stakeholders.

REFERENCE

1. National Quality Forum. Creating a framework to support measure development for telehealth. August 31, 2017. **https://www.qualityforum.org/Publications/2017/08/Creating_a_Framework_to_Support_Measure_Development_for_Telehealth.aspx**. Accessed May 13, 2021.

CHAPTER 12
Determining Methods to Retrieve Data for Telehealth Services

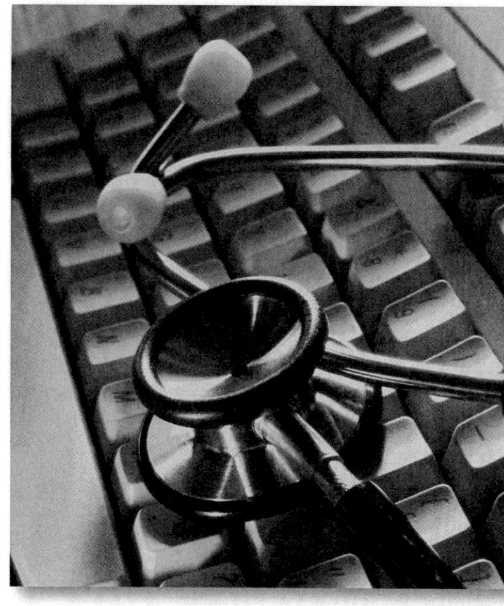

As highlighted in Chapter 11, when developing metrics to track for a service, it is important to understand your organization's priorities and focus. Are there specific initiatives going on within your organization that your pharmacy service could demonstrate impact? Are there upcoming strategic priorities that could leverage pharmacy telehealth practice? How is your organization aligned with reimbursement and future strategy for reimbursement? And the most important question: where do we find the information?

Breaking down metrics into different categories may be helpful when determining where to find the information you will need to measure outcomes. Clinical data will likely always be obtained through the electronic health record. Financial data may come from a variety of sources, depending on which metrics you are tracking. If you are tracking measures that are more closely related to value-based care, you may need to engage your population health partners or other teams that are involved in value-based care. Look for quality committees, clinically integrated network teams, or even a clinic manager to help determine where they may obtain data. For revenue-based measures, your electronic health record may offer some reporting capabilities. Your clinic manager may also be a resource to help you obtain these data. If you are in a larger health system, you may have a finance manager who can help gather these data.

Patient and provider experience outcomes may come from sources external to the electronic health record. The method for finding patient experience outcomes will largely depend on how you elect to track patient experience. Utilization of tools that are used throughout your clinic or health system will likely require partnership with the clinic manager or physician group/health-system leadership. If you are using a self-developed tool, data access and tracking are easier. Provider experiences with pharmacy services will likely need to be a tool that is developed and tracked internally. While there is not a wealth of literature published on provider satisfaction with telehealth pharmacy services, some papers outline provider perception and/or satisfaction with pharmacy services in general. Albanese and colleagues described creating a survey to measure provider perception of pharmacy services within a patient-centered medical home (PCMH).[1] They developed a 63-item survey to determine which pharmacy services were worthwhile when considering clinical, cost and medication access, and educational services. The survey was administered using an online platform and included physicians, nurse practitioners, and physician assistants at the primary care PCMH. Through use of this survey, Albanese et al. were able to identify specific pharmacy services that the providers considered to be of the most value, including medication counseling, polypharmacy assessment,

DOI 10.37573/9781585286928.012

medication adherence assessment, and medication reconciliation.[1] In addition, in the primary care setting, pharmacists have been found to reduce burnout among primary care providers and benefit patient care in multiple areas, including satisfaction that patients were receiving better care, increased provider access, and achievement of quality measures.[2]

Tool for telehealth pharmacy practice evaluation: Data mining and analysis is a fluid and dynamic process that usually involves key stakeholders across an organization. It may be challenging to engage all the necessary parties initially, so have patience! Also, be aware of how upgrades to electronic health record platforms may impact metric reporting.

HOW TO TRACK METRICS

When determining how to track metrics, it is important to understand what organizational resources you may have available to you. If you are a pharmacist within an independent physician practice, it may be harder to leverage reports and data retrieval from the electronic health record in an automated fashion. If you are part of a larger health system with a robust physician group network, however, you may be able to leverage data analysts or Information Systems (IS) resources to help with metric tracking via reports and dashboards.

Many organizations start tracking service metrics with homegrown tools, such as databases or spreadsheets. If your organization takes this approach, it is important to standardize components of the tracking when possible. For example, if the same service is provided at multiple physician clinics, it would be important to have a spreadsheet template that is used to track the same data points everywhere the service is provided. This allows for the data to be uniform and easier to analyze for the service overall.

Examples for Tracking Different Types of Metrics for Pharmacy Telehealth Practice

Chapter 11 highlighted multiple metrics across five different domains used for pharmacy telehealth practice. This chapter provides some meaningful examples demonstrating the application of some of those metrics.

Access to Care

In many areas of the country, access to a primary care provider is delayed due to a shortage of primary care providers. Over 7,200 primary care healthcare professional shortage areas (HPSAs) have been designated across the United States by the Health Resources and Services Administration (HRSA) in the U.S. Department of Health and Human Services.[3] This can contribute to patients delaying or not receiving needed care.

Ambulatory care pharmacists delivering care through telehealth technologies can help bridge the care gap in HPSAs and increase available primary care access through collaboration with providers. Tracking and evaluating key access metrics can describe that value. Demonstrating a decrease in median lag time or third next available appointment can serve as valuable metrics in support for ambulatory care pharmacy services. If a provider is able to increase their panel size through partnership with a pharmacist, more patients receive needed care.

A 2017 study by Brunisholz and colleagues[4] evaluated the quality of team-based care in patients with diabetes or high blood pressure with or without an ambulatory care pharmacist on the care team. Care delivered by the pharmacist was provided both face-to-face and over the telephone, with about 70% of encounters delivered remotely. Study results demonstrated increased touches with the clinical care team in the cohort with the pharmacist on the team (8.4 vs. 5.1 visits per patient-year, $p < 0.001$). The authors hypothesized that more frequent follow-up was a contributing factor to the positive clinical outcomes that were achieved. Leveraging telehealth to deliver care allowed the pharmacists to increase patient touches and ultimately improve care.[4]

Financial Impact/Cost

Metrics demonstrating increased revenue or expense savings can prove valuable to building and sustaining any ambulatory care model, including telehealth pharmacy practice services. Understanding the priorities and focus of an organization will be key to determining which financial metrics might be most impactful. For example, in an integrated health system highly focused in value-based care, demonstrating a decrease in per member per month (PMPM) expenses might be a key metric. A private practice in a fee-for-service model may prioritize the profit generated per encounter.

Financial impact on patients, payers, and the health system are all important considerations. Reducing patient out-of-pocket expense for medications, for example, can result in positive patient experiences, improve medication adherence, and reduce provider frustrations. Payers are interested in any demonstration of decreased expenses (medical or pharmaceutical). Tracking and reporting improvements in generic prescribing, formulary adherence, or PMPM will be valuable metrics to gain support for one's telehealth service. Return on investment (ROI) may be a difficult metric to obtain, depending on data accessibility, but it will speak loudly to decision makers within most organizations. An example of a simple spreadsheet used to track financial metrics is provided in **Figure 12.1**.

Hawes and colleagues studied the financial outcomes of pharmacist-led telehealth visits for both diabetes management and warfarin management. Services were billed using incident-to billing with a supervising physician. For anticoagulation management, G0248 was billed once for training, and future e-visits were billed once monthly using CPT code 99444. In the diabetes group, e-visits were billed using CPT code 99444. The margin per patient for the anticoagulation program was estimated to be $25 per month for the first year and $16 per month for the second year. The margin per patient for the diabetes program was estimated to be $25 per month, based on an average of 2.4 e-visits and 1.4 in-person visits over four months. This study helped demonstrate that there are opportunities to generate reimbursement from telehealth pharmacy practice visits with a positive net margin.[5]

Patient Name (Last, First)	Doctor (Full Name)	Time Spent (mins)	Inpatient readmission w/in 30 days (Y/N)	Planned inpatient Readmission	Rx's transferred in	ED Visit w/in 30 days (without an inpatient admission)	Number or contacts	Money Saved Per Month	Transferred out
Patient 1	MD1	15			11		1	$ 623	
Patient 2	MD2	20			2		1	$ 160	
Patient 3	MD5	15			5		1	$ 124	
Patient 4	MD6	45			20		4		
Patient 5	MD3	15			4		1	$ 40	
Patient 6	MD7	40					2	$ 95	
Patient 7	MD5				16		1	$ 504	
Patient 8	MD8	10			3		2		
Patient 9	MD3	15			3		1	$ 52	
Patient 10	MD3	30			1		2	$ 190	
Patient 11	MD5	15					1		
Patient 12	MD5	30			10		1	$ 172	
Patient 13	MD6				7		1	$ 22	
Patient 14	MD4	30					8		
Patient 15	MD6						1	$ 59	
Patient 16	MD7	20			1		1	$ 45	
Totals			0	0	83	0	29	$ 2,086	0
Averages		23					2	$ 174	

Figure 12.1. Financial metric tracking spreadsheet

Experience

There is a lot of emphasis on patient experience within hospitals and health systems. Consider the following example from a clinical ambulatory pharmacist in a transplant clinic. Two surgeons worked with the solid organ transplant service. One had the best results following surgery, but a terrible bedside manner. A second surgeon had a higher complication and failure rate than the first but was very personable at the bedside. Which surgeon do you think patients perceived delivered the higher quality of care? That's right, surgeon number two. Providing a quality patient experience is vital to the perceived quality of care and loyalty to the health system and care team.

When considering how to evaluate patient experience or patient satisfaction with a service, it is a good idea to see what methods for gauging patient experience your organization already leverages. You may be able to utilize a platform that is already in place and will require little manual work. Another benefit to using a preexisting patient experience platform is that organizational leadership will already be familiar with the tool, so it will require little explaining or teaching. A downside to using a preexisting tool is that the questions may not all be relevant to pharmacy services, or it may not capture specific questions that you wish to address. For example, pharmacists at one health system on the East Coast adapted the survey used for medical practices, creating a pharmacist clinical survey. This provided valuable insight into patient experience with the care being delivered by clinical pharmacists. As an adapted survey, it also included some questions that were not directly related to the patient's experience seeing the pharmacist (e.g., nurse/medical assistant support). Further adaptation of a survey tool to address the uniqueness of a telehealth service may also be needed.

Hatton and colleagues published a study in 2018 evaluating the patient experience with pharmacist-provided care using clinical video telehealth (CVT). For the purpose of this study, *telehealth* was defined as video-teleconferencing. The researchers hypothesized that patient satisfaction would not differ between face-to-face delivery and care provided using CVT. Patients were asked to answer 10 questions assessing the pharmacist's patient-centered communication and clinical competence and skills. The survey was self-administered. Survey questions utilized a typical 5-point Likert Scale for responses, with a score of 1 indicating a high level of disagreement with the statement and a level of 5 indicating a high level of agreement. Baseline demographics were similar between face-to-face and CVT populations. A response rate for the survey was not tracked. Based on the survey results, greater than 80% of patients in both the face-to-face and CVT populations responded with high agreement or satisfaction (a Likert score of 5) with the pharmacist use of patient-centered communication as well as clinical competence and skills. There were no statistically significant differences between the two groups. This led the authors to conclude that patient satisfaction did not differ based on the care delivery method.[6]

A 2016 article by Maxwell and associates assessed patient satisfaction with a pharmacist-led CVT program for chronic disease management. A clinical pharmacy specialist (CPS) provided clinical services via CVT to patients at a clinic where there were no onsite clinical pharmacy services. Patient satisfaction with the care provided by the pharmacist and CVT as a care delivery method was assessed as a secondary outcome. Twenty-six patients received services during the six-month evaluation period. A modified version of the Satisfaction with Pharmacists (SWiP) Scale was used, with three questions added to assess patient satisfaction with services delivered via CVT. The survey used a 5-point Likert Scale to measure responses, with a zero indicating that a patient was not at all satisfied with services and a 4 indicating patients were very satisfied with services. All 26 patients completing six months of pharmacy services delivered via CVT completed the survey. The median score was 39.5 (interquartile range 36–40) with a maximum score of 40. When looking specifically at the questions related to CVT as a method of care delivery, the median CVT satisfaction score was 12 (interquartile range 12–12) with a maximum score of 12. These results led the authors to conclude that patient satisfaction with CVT as a care delivery method was very high.[7]

If leveraging a preexisting patient satisfaction tool within your health system isn't possible, there is always the option to develop your own tool. Options may include a brief comment-card-style survey where patients may answer a few questions and then have a place for open comments or feedback. Comment cards can be mailed with a self-addressed stamped envelope provided for return. Another option would be to develop a brief phone survey that can be administered within several days of an appointment. With this option, it is important that the survey be short, with a rating scale that is easy for patients to follow over the phone. With all of these options, maintaining the patient's sense of anonymity is important. Patients may be more likely to provide open and honest feedback if they have a sense of anonymity. For example, with a phone survey, it is likely best if the pharmacist who performed the service is not the individual to reach out to the patient to collect data. This might be a role for another pharmacist on the team or a great way to leverage students within a layered learning model.

Effectiveness

As outlined in Chapter 11, measures of effectiveness relate specifically to patient outcomes and often may be clinical markers of disease improvement or assessment of healthcare utilization. Following is an outline of several published studies demonstrating the effectiveness of telehealth services. A more in-depth review of published telehealth literature and positive outcomes can be found in Chapter 1 of the present volume.

The aforementioned study conducted by Brunisholz et al.[4] demonstrated positive clinical outcomes, utilizing recognized disease markers as the metrics. In this study, an estimated 70% of patient encounters were conducted virtually. Patients in the pharmacist cohort were more likely to achieve their HbA1c and/or blood pressure goals when a pharmacist was part of the care team. Additionally, these targets were met more rapidly than with the usual care cohort. Kaplan-Meier survival analysis showed improved achievement of goals at 180 days postintervention (48% vs. 27%, $p < 0.001$ meeting blood pressure targets; 39% vs. 30%, $p < 0.05$ meeting diabetes targets).[4]

A systematic review and meta-analysis reviewed the effectiveness of pharmacy telehealth services. The review found that most services were for chronic disease management, with the telephone being the most common mode of communication. This review found an overall positive impact on outcomes related to chronic disease management.[8]

A study by Litke et al. looked at both telephone and video encounters in which chronic disease management was provided for rural veterans. In this study, comprehensive medication management was provided by clinical pharmacy specialists via both telephonic and telehealth pharmacy practice models. Statistically significant improvements in diabetes and hypertension, as well as clinical improvements in lipid management and tobacco cessation, were seen.[9]

There is not a considerable breadth of literature describing the success of clinical pharmacy services provided via telehealth compared with traditional methods. In addition, emerging telehealth technologies, including remote patient monitoring devices, create ample opportunities for pharmacists to engage in practice-based research to add to the literature.

Utilization

When evaluating utilization of a service, several options can be considered. One could look at the potential number of patients eligible for a service and how many of those engage in the service. That could be further broken down to look at those that may only engage in an initial visit versus those who engage in follow-up visits. If your engagement in a service is low, it may be worthwhile to reach out to patients who did not engage at all to determine barriers to engagement. You could also follow up with patients who only had one visit and no follow-up visits to help determine why the individual did not find value in the service. Chapter 14. will discuss more in-depth barriers to patient utilization of telehealth pharmacy services.

Tool for telehealth pharmacy practice evaluation: Establish metrics and methods for data collection prior to the start of a service! The metrics and tracking methods should be reevaluated on a periodic basis to ensure that the metrics being measured are still relevant and that the data collection methods are as efficient as possible.

REFERENCES

1. Albanese NP, Pignato AM, Monte SV. Provider perception of pharmacy services in the patient-centered medical home. *J Pharm Pract.* 2017 Dec;30(6):612-620. doi: 10.1177/0897190016679759.
2. Funk KA, Pestka DL, Roth McClurg MT, et al. Primary care providers believe that comprehensive medication management improves their work-life. *J Am Board Fam Med.* 2019; 32(4):462-473. doi: 10.3122/jabfm.2019.04.180376.
3. Designated Health Professional Shortage Areas Statistics: Designated HPSA Quarterly Summary. Bureau of Health Workforce, Health Resources and Services Administration (HRSA), U.S. Department of Health and Human Services. **https://data.hrsa.gov/topics/health-workforce/shortage-areas**. Accessed May 18, 2021.
4. Brunisholz KD, Olson JL, Anderson JW, et al. "Pharming out" support: A promising approach to integrating clinical pharmacists into established primary care medical home practices. *J Int Med Res.* 2018 Jan;46(1):234-248. doi: 10.3399/bjgp19X705461.
5. Hawes EM, Lamber E, Reid A, et al. Implementation and evaluation of a pharmacist-led electronic visit program for diabetes and anticoagulation care in a patient-centered medical home. *Am J Health Syst Pharm.* 2018 Jun 15;75(12):901-910. doi: 10.2146/ajhp170174.
6. Hatton J, Chandra R, Lucius D, et al. Patient satisfaction of pharmacist-provided care via clinical video teleconferencing. *J Pharm Pract.* October 2018;31(5):429-433. doi: 10.1177/0897190017715561.
7. Maxwell LG, McFarland MS, Baker JW, et al. Evaluation of the impact of a pharmacist-led telehealth clinic on diabetes-related goals of therapy in a veteran population. *Pharmacotherapy.* March 2016;36(3):348-356. doi: 10.1002/phar.1719.
8. Niznik JD, He H, Kane-Gill SL. Impact of clinical pharmacist services delivered via telemedicine in the outpatient or ambulatory care setting: A systematic review. *Res Social Adm Pharm.* 2018 Aug;14(8):707-717. doi: 10.1016/j.sapharm.2017.10.011.
9. Litke J, Spoutz L, Ahlstorm D, et al. Impact of the clinical pharmacy specialist in telehealth primary care. *Am J Health Syst Pharm.* July 1, 2018;75(13):982-986. doi: 10.2146/ajhp170633.

CHAPTER 13 Methods for Sharing Metrics

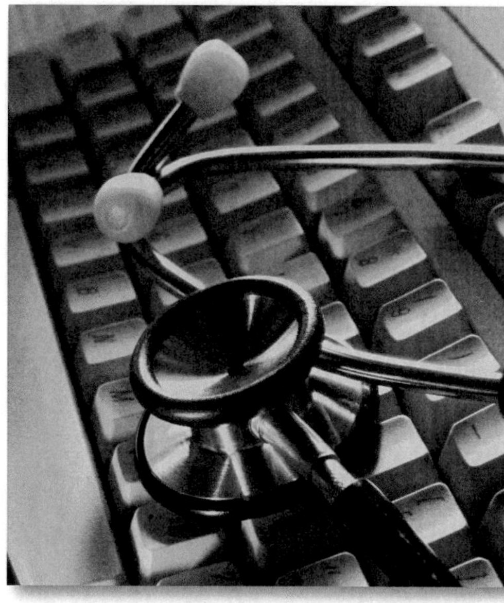

After identifying meaningful metrics that demonstrate the value of a telehealth pharmacy service and the pharmacists delivering the service, determining a strategy to share the results is important. Without sharing the metrics with leaders, their value and the effort expended to track the data will be wasted. As you prepare to share metrics within your organization, it is vital to identify those individuals who need to receive the communication. Consider key stakeholders such as departmental leaders within the pharmacy department, physicians' group, or health system. You may also consider sharing data at the individual clinic level—sharing with office leadership and providers. If your organization has a telehealth or virtual health division, sharing your data with this team will also be meaningful. Outlining the timing and methods for sharing the data are also key considerations. Sharing data can demonstrate the success of a service and help spur further growth of the service.

DASHBOARDS

A dashboard is a valuable tool to track, display, and share pertinent data. A dashboard provides a graphical representation of priority metrics that can be reviewed and digested at a glance. Dashboards are an effective means of communicating priority data to multiple groups. Managers can use them to share priorities and progress with their employees. They can also use them to communicate key metrics and progress to supervisors and even the executive-level leaders within a company, often referred to as C-suite due to titles. With thoughtful selection of the most important metrics, the same dashboard will be meaningful for both those on the front line and those with decision-making responsibilities.

Like identifying the right metrics, considering how your organization digests and displays data will be an important consideration when you are developing a dashboard. Focusing on key performance indicators (KPI) and those metrics that most clearly display the productivity and impact of ambulatory care is important when caring for patients virtually.

At Intermountain Healthcare based in Salt Lake City, Utah, a digital dashboard was created to display KPI for ambulatory care pharmacists (**Figure 13.1**). These pharmacists document encounters in the electronic health record, including key information about time spent with the patient, type of encounter (e.g., telehealth, face-to-face), and medication therapy problems identified and addressed. These data are drawn into the dashboard directly from the electronic data warehouse. Ambulatory care pharmacists, managers, and administrators can all access the dashboard at any time to view data. Continuous improvement efforts are reviewed and tracked using the digital dashboard. Managers and administrators

DOI 10.37573/9781585286928.013

Amcare Intervention Summary

Date Range: YTD
Start Date: 11/3/2020
End Date: 11/3/2020
Last Updated: 4/12/2021 8:09:23 AM
Pharmacist: (All)
At Risk: (All)

	Total Interactions	Interactions/Pharm	Avg ..Time/Interactions ...	Total Telehealth	Total Phone	Total Electronic	Total Video	Total In-Person	Total MTPs	MTPs PharmD	Total Actions	Actions PharmD	Total Unique Patients	Total Time Hrs
January 2021	1,655	103	24	1,456	1,079	360	17	189	1,863	116	2,718	170	1,230	657.38
February 2021	1,531	85	24	1,357	1,012	336	9	167	1,798	100	2,554	142	1,129	595.53
March 2021	2,099	91	24	1,827	1,368	442	17	256	2,513	109	3,620	157	1,453	839.36
April 2021	583	31	22	[illegible]	[illegible]	117	8	82	676	36	996	52	522	214.82
Grand Total	5,868	245	24	[illegible]	[illegible]	1,255	51	694	6,850	285	9,888	412	3,000	2,307.09

Month, Year of PERF_MONDATE: **March 2021**
Total Telehealth: **1,827**

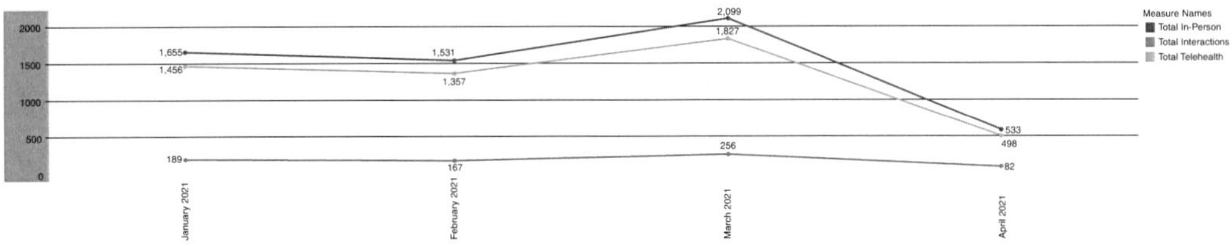

Amcare Intervention Summary

PHARMACIST	Total Unique Patients	Total Interactions	Total Time Hrs	Avg Time Interactions Min	Total In-Person	Total Telehealth	Total Phone	Total Electronic	Total Video	Total Null	Total MTPs	Total Actions	Actions Interaction	Actions Hour
	244	524	186.44	21	34	487	414	71	2	3	450	853	1.6	4.58
	6	6	0.93	11	5	1	0	0	1	0	0	7	1.2	7.53
	22	26	2.50	6	16	9	8	0	1	1	23	48	1.8	19.20
	355	599	183.57	19	50	547	436	107	4	2	320	846	1.4	4.61
	5	5	3.34	40	5	0	0	0	0	0	2	6	1.2	1.80
	23	24	13.07	34	2	21	17	4	0	1	36	40	1.7	3.06
	118	154	88.33	34	48	106	85	21	0	0	207	331	2.1	3.75
	103	159	117.90	45	0	158	93	65	0	1	201	240	1.5	2.04
	377	754	277.06	22	23	728	537	191	0	3	784	1,492	2.0	5.39
	70	139	83.79	37	38	94	80	13	1	7	183	246	1.8	2.94
	128	173	34.38	13	158	8	4	4	0	7	82	84	0.5	2.41
	35	46	16.59	22	5	41	40	0	1	0	41	103	2.2	6.21
	412	533	148.07	17	24	509	323	186	0	0	607	790	1.5	5.34
	79	257	167.09	40	1	249	159	82	8	7	458	547	2.1	3.27
	273	674	226.02	20	2	671	467	203	1	1	1,082	1,242	1.8	5.50
	21	21	6.09	24	4	17	17	0	0	0	19	26	1.2	4.27
	1	1	0.17	10	0	1	1	0	0	0	2	2	2.0	11.76
	1	1	0.08	5	0	1	1	0	0	0	0	2	2.0	25.00
	82	158	65.04	25	5	153	149	2	2	0	177	371	2.3	5.70
	169	424	176.56	25	46	377	349	28	0	1	369	493	1.2	2.79
	7	8	3.75	28	7	1	1	0	0	0	6	16	2.0	4.27
	372	829	325.96	24	129	699	480	204	15	1	1,298	1,465	1.8	4.49
	21	35	20.62	35	4	31	31	0	0	0	40	89	2.5	4.32
	153	318	159.72	30	88	229	140	74	15	1	463	549	1.7	3.44
Grand Total	3,000	5,868	2,307.09	24	694	5,138	3,832	1,255	51	36	6,850	9,888	1.7	4.29

RFI	Total In-Person	Total Phone	Total Electronic	Total Video	Total Telehealth	Total Null	Total MTPs	Total Actions	Avg Time/Interactions Min
Null	4	21	7	1	29	18	28	54	
Comprehensive Med Review	182	122	16	6	144	0	494	572	42
CPA - Anticoag	9	85	105	0	190	1	152	288	13
CPA - DM	378	2,065	324	34	2,423	8	3,511	4,855	25
CPA - HTN	27	366	34	0	400	0	372	671	21
Disease state management	78	789	491	5	1,285	6	1,492	2,277	18
Drug information question	10	98	246	0	344	1	347	457	19
Pain management	2	18	11	4	33	0	30	52	22
Transition of Care	4	268	21	1	290	2	424	662	36
Grand Total	694	3,832	1,255	51	5,138	36	6,850	9,888	24

Figure 13.1. Ambulatory care dashboard example

use data from the dashboard to help document the value and productivity of ambulatory care pharmacists.

A fully digitized dashboard will likely not be your first step. Starting somewhere is important. If all you can do is track data in a spreadsheet and highlight a couple of metrics, it is worth showcasing that effort. The current version of the Intermountain ambulatory care dashboard is not where it started. Multiple iterations of the dashboard were tried before arriving at the current version.

Depending on the size of your organization, ambulatory care pharmacy team, and availability of information systems (IS) resources, an automated dashboard may not be feasible. Many ambulatory pharmacists or small ambulatory teams that are beginning services may find it easier to leverage spreadsheets and database tools when first starting. These platforms typically offer many tools for data manipulation and analysis. These strategies can also be standardized. If more than one pharmacist is providing the service, this will allow the same data to be collected across pharmacists and locations.

Once the data are analyzed, it can be presented using other methods such as slides or one-page summaries. Consider what control group your data could be compared to in order to demonstrate impact. For example, will you make a comparison to baseline patient data or standard of

Box 13.1. Potential Data Collection and Analysis Tools

- Spreadsheet programs
- Database programs
- REDCap (Research Electronic Data Capture)
- Data analysis programs

care? A downside of manual data collection and analysis is that it does have a built-in delay and is not available in real time as an automated dashboard would be. Even with standardization, there is the possibility that data may not be recorded in the same way or that there may be gaps in the data requiring manual look-up. It also can be very time consuming for pharmacists to complete and may decrease the top-of-license activities they are able to perform. **Box 13.1** lists various options for data collection and analysis.

Tool for telehealth pharmacy practice evaluation: A dashboard is ideal for data collection and display of metrics. Many services do not start out with a dashboard but leverage home-grown tools early on.

PATIENT STORIES

Never underestimate the impact of a powerful patient story. Data demonstrating success with clinics' outcomes or financial wins are important. Layering in real stories about how pharmacists positively impact the lives of patients can be very powerful. The emotional pull of the stories coupled with positive data can be very persuasive.

You should identify patient success stories that are part of your telehealth pharmacy program. Storytelling can help demonstrate the success of your program and build support for continuing or expanding. Storytelling makes your data more real and more personal. It can evoke emotion.

Storytelling can occur in a variety of ways. It can be in the form of one to two patient vignettes to describe the success of your program. Alternatively, it can comprise several statements from the patient to demonstrate the importance of the service from the patient's perspective. Some organizations may also look to use a digital approach—making videos or posts on social media to highlight patient success stories. Sharing these stories with key stakeholders can create a ripple effect of sharing those stories throughout the organization.

Communication with the C-Suite

When communicating with the C-suite, it is important to understand what metrics and stories are going to have the greatest resonance. This is where having that understanding of organizational priorities, strategic planning, and reimbursement strategy is critical. The C-suite likely doesn't need to hear all the metrics that are being tracked for a service—just those that align most closely with organizational priorities to make the information meaningful. Another consideration when communicating with the C-suite is to keep information concise. Provide the most relevant metrics and outcomes. Contemplate adding a patient success story or two. Be sure not to overload the C-suite with data and information. If you do not limit your information, the key points may be missed, and attention will be shifted to less important details. Consider limiting materials to a one-page handout or a handful of presentation slides. Use charts and tables when possible and limit the amount of text. If you have a dashboard that your C-suite has access to, providing the information to access that dashboard and the most relevant pieces is also important.

Often in healthcare organizations, physicians are a driving force behind the direction a healthcare system may take. Aligning your telehealth pharmacy practice service with a physician champion can be beneficial, especially if that individual can provide support within C-suite conversations. A physician champion may be able to provide you with insight into what metrics could be most relevant to the organization and also provide information on barriers you may encounter as you seek to use metrics and outcomes to continue or scale work within an organization.

Scaling the Work within an Organization

The disruption of the pandemic in 2020 propelled advancement of telehealth throughout healthcare. Continuing that advancement within ambulatory care pharmacy services requires an understanding of pharmacist productivity. Metrics are key to scaling your telehealth pharmacy practice service. They can help you understand what can be expected from each pharmacist. For example, a metric showing average time per patient encounter can inform how many patients a pharmacist could care for during a shift. Whether it is the amount of time per patient encounter or estimating a panel size of patients that a pharmacist could provide care for, it is important to have these estimates available when you are considering service expansion. This can help determine how many full-time equivalents (FTEs) would be needed to launch a service whether across several locations or across the health system.

When considering when and how to scale work throughout the organization, reviewing utilization patterns of existing resources can also be important. For example, do all existing pharmacists have a full schedule, or do some pharmacists have schedules that may be only 70% full or less? That open time may be able to be leveraged to support telehealth services for patients in another clinic location. In addition, looking at lead time for a new appointment slot for patients is another marker that can help determine existing capacity and potential for enlarging patient panel size. It is important that data reporting can provide this information in order to best determine a strategy for scaling services.

CHAPTER 14 Anticipating and Overcoming Barriers

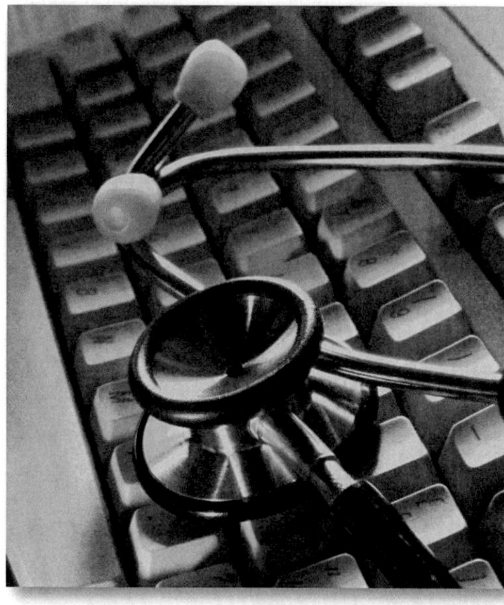

In the journey to determine, define, and track metrics when starting a service or measuring an already existing service, there are going to be barriers along the way. Being able to anticipate these barriers ahead of time can lead to less frustration and more success.

IDENTIFYING WHICH METRICS ARE MOST MEANINGFUL TO YOUR ORGANIZATION

As we discussed in previous chapters, being able to align metrics with organizational priorities is critical. Selecting metrics that matter to your organization will make it more likely that positive outcomes will hold weight with leadership within your organization, but this selection may be challenging. If you are in a larger health system, look to leadership to identify what may be important. It could be pharmacy leadership, physician's group leadership, quality leadership, or leadership in the population health or value-based care space. These individuals will have knowledge about the organization's strategies for reimbursement and for providing care. Clinic managers can also be a great starting point for gaining insight into metrics that are important to the organization. Clinic managers are often responsible for sharing quality data with providers and will likely have insight into financial data and reimbursement strategy as well. Identifying potential key stakeholders up front that you can engage to learn about what quality metrics would be important to your organization is critical.

LEVERAGING INFORMATION SYSTEM RESOURCES

In many organizations, whether a private practice office or a physician's group in a large health system, information system (IS) resources are often difficult to come by. Understanding the structure of your organization's IS team may help you leverage resources. Generally, a particular subset of the IS team supports an organization's electronic health record. Within that subset, there may be additional smaller teams that support specific areas of the electronic health record. Some organizations may have virtual health teams, pharmacy teams, and/or ambulatory teams for their electronic health record. One or more of these teams may be able to offer support for tracking of selected metrics.

When possible, it is ideal to capture data needed for metric tracking within the documentation template. This creates less work for the pharmacist(s) if double documentation can be avoided. Some electronic health record platforms offer customizable forms in which data can be selected or captured via a comment box. Other options might include the use of specific "smart" statements put into clinical documentation and later pulled into a report.

DOI 10.37573/9781585286928.014

Some of the options described above reflect the ideal state in leveraging IS resources for more automated reporting. As discussed in earlier chapters, some organizations or practices may not be able to achieve this ideal early on in pharmacy services or with pilot projects. It may be necessary to employ other tools (described above in Box 13.1) to track metric data. If you are unsure as to which types of tools may be available within your organization, your IS team will be able to help with that as well. Alternative options may be available that could support data collection for metric tracking.

Financial Transparency

When discussing data collection for metric tracking, it may not always be feasible to access the data you need. Depending on your position within an organization and the organization's stance on sharing financial information, access to some financial data may be limited. This could be a large barrier if you belong to an organization that is more focused on fee-for-service, for it will limit the ability to assess the financial sustainability of the service.

If you have access to financial data, it is important to ensure that you have access to the data you need for any metrics you select. For example, if you are in an organization that is part of an Accountable Care Organization (ACO), having access to ACO patients' cost of care would be important. Depending on what financial metrics you may be tracking, it can still be difficult—even with access to data. Identifying revenue can be straightforward, especially if your electronic health record identifies a service provider. This service provider can be the pharmacist for any pharmacist-provided service, even if it is billed incident-to. This can allow for tracking billing codes and attached revenue for any services with the pharmacist as the service provider. Some organizations elect to use tracking codes, which are specific codes created by an organization to track visits completed by a pharmacist. These codes can be added to visits with billable charges to separate those claims tied to pharmacy services. Other organizations may elect to create specific visit types for tracking pharmacy-specific visits and services.

Financial incentives tied to value-based care models may be more difficult to track. Understanding any value-based care models your organization may be engaged in is very important for both establishing and tracking these metrics to ensure you can attribute improvement in quality measures and closures in care gaps to pharmacists performing services that align with these quality measures.

When identifying and selecting metrics to track, financial metrics may be the most challenging for several reasons. Access to financial data can be a barrier. Even in circumstances where you have access to the necessary data, being able to attribute that financial benefit to the pharmacist can be a struggle. Proactively working to understand what data you might have access to and how data flows within your health system and with third-party payers is important. Developing a solid strategy can help ensure that pharmacists receive the appropriate attribution for the services they are providing.

Tool for telehealth pharmacy practice evaluation: Brainstorming for barriers or challenges to determining metrics and tracking data for telehealth pharmacy services can help with preparation to overcome these obstacles. One of the most challenging barriers for many pharmacists is transparency related to financial metrics. Before establishing financial metrics to measure, involve key stakeholders from the finance department or clinic leadership to determine what data will be available to track and measure.

PATIENT EXPERIENCE

Having a strong workflow to help patients navigate their telehealth experience is important. A 2020 systematic review and meta-analysis shared the top patient-reported barriers to leveraging telehealth in older adults (Kruse et al. 2020).[1] These themes of patient-reported barriers are listed

Box 14.1. Themes of Patient-Reported Barriers to Accessing Telehealth

- Technical literacy
- Lack of desire
- Cost
- Lack of technical support
- Visual acuity
- Social implications
- Ownership of technology
- Privacy and security
- Medical literacy
- Trust of the Internet
- Mental acuity
- Hand–eye coordination
- Auditory acuity
- Computer anxiety

Source: Adapted from Kruse C, Fohn J, Wilson N, et al. *JMIR Med Inform.* August 12, 2020;8(8):e20359.

in **Box 14.1**. Being able to address some of these barriers may help improve the patient experience. For example, can your organization provide additional support for patients to help them navigate telehealth technologies? Does your organization offer the ability for patients to gain access to devices to support telehealth, potentially through grant-funded programs? Could your organization provide education to patients on the safety and security of telehealth platforms and telehealth encounters? Are you able to provide a demonstration of a telehealth visit for a patient while they are in the office? Are there specific platforms that may address the visual or auditory needs of patients?

If your clinic or your organization has a way to proactively address some of these themes of patient-reported barriers to accessing telehealth, it may help increase your overall engagement in telehealth services as well as patient experience. It is important to review the feedback you receive regarding the patient experience to see what barriers may exist for your specific populations.

PATIENT SAFETY

Patient safety concerns are still present with telehealth services and require some different advance preparation. The Agency for Healthcare Research and Quality (AHRQ) published an article outlining various considerations for patient safety and telehealth during the pandemic, but some of these considerations may extend beyond the pandemic as long as we continue telehealth pharmacy practice services.[2]

Telehealth offers the opportunity to provide a new way for patients to access care that may be more convenient for them. During a pandemic, it also may be safer for patients to engage in services via telehealth instead of traditional methods. Even outside of a pandemic, telehealth offers flexibility to engage patients who may have transportation issues or live far from the clinic, or high-risk patients who may benefit from telehealth visits to avoid potential exposures. Telehealth visits are not always appropriate for patients. Workflows designed to identify which patients may be more appropriate for in-person visits and when to advance to in-person care are critical.

Modalities for reporting patient safety events should be available. The ability to track events related to telehealth services versus traditional services may be important. It will help medication safety teams identify specific patterns with telehealth services that could be addressed from a system perspective to improve patient safety. These events can be learning opportunities for teams and for the healthcare system seeking to improve processes.

REFERENCES

1. Kruse C, Fohn J, Wilson N, et al. Utilization barriers and medical outcomes commensurate with the use of telehealth among older adults: Systematic review. *JMIR Med Inform*. August 12, 2020;8(8):e20359. doi: 10.2196/20359.
2. Telehealth and Patient Safety during the COVID-19 Response. Agency for Healthcare Research and Quality (AHRQ). **https://psnet.ahrq.gov/perspective/telehealth-and-patient-safety-during-covid-19-response**. Accessed May 18, 2021.

SECTION 4: CLINICAL VIGNETTE

Scenario 1

You are working on selecting key metrics to track and report on for your telehealth pharmacy services. Your clinic has been very focused on how the pharmacist can improve the clinical outcomes of patients. At the current time, your clinic is not involved in any value-based care plans, but there is talk about partnering with a local employer-sponsored health plan to improve patient outcomes specifically related to diabetes. While revenue generation has not been a focus of your position, you have heard rumblings recently about a renewed focus on clinic revenue and improving margins. What metrics might be ideal for you to track based on this information?

Response 1

Clinical outcomes of patients with diabetes would be a key metric to focus on given the information above. Capturing information related to hemoglobin A1c (HbA1c), statin use, blood pressure control, nephropathy screening, and eye exams would be important. Also consider how you will demonstrate changes in these measures. Will you compare to patient's baseline data or create a standard of care group for comparison?

In addition to the metrics above, you will also want to ensure that you are tracking revenue generated from your chronic care management (CCM) billing. Even if revenue is not something that pharmacy services have been asked to generate in the past, creating a financially sustainable service is crucial. In this case, the physician practice is not involved in value-based care, so generating and tracking revenue is an important consideration.

Scenario 2

You are creating a presentation reviewing metrics to share with your clinic leadership, including providers, to demonstrate the successes to date of telehealth pharmacy services. You feel that your data set is very compelling, but you are hoping to make it more humane to allow your audience to connect to the service and patients on an emotional level. You decide to include a brief patient success story to share with the audience but are struggling with how much detail to provide or what type of success to demonstrate.

Response 2

Including a patient success story can create an emotional response in your audience that will lay a strong foundation for receiving the data to be presented. Patient success stories do not have to be long or involved. A short vignette can be very powerful. After consideration, you decide to include the following patient story for a patient who received telehealth pharmacy services. "A patient was referred to pharmacy due to uncontrolled diabetes, which was putting him in jeopardy of losing **his** CDL license. His initial hemoglobin A1c (HbA1c) was 9.9%. Following medication adjustments and lifestyle education, this patient's HbA1c was reduced to 6.9% six weeks after initial pharmacy appointment. Pharmacy continued to follow the patient, and three months later his HbA1c reduction was maintained at 6.5%. During this time, the patient also had a 5% reduction in body weight. This patient was able to maintain his CDL and keep his job with the support he received via telehealth pharmacy services."

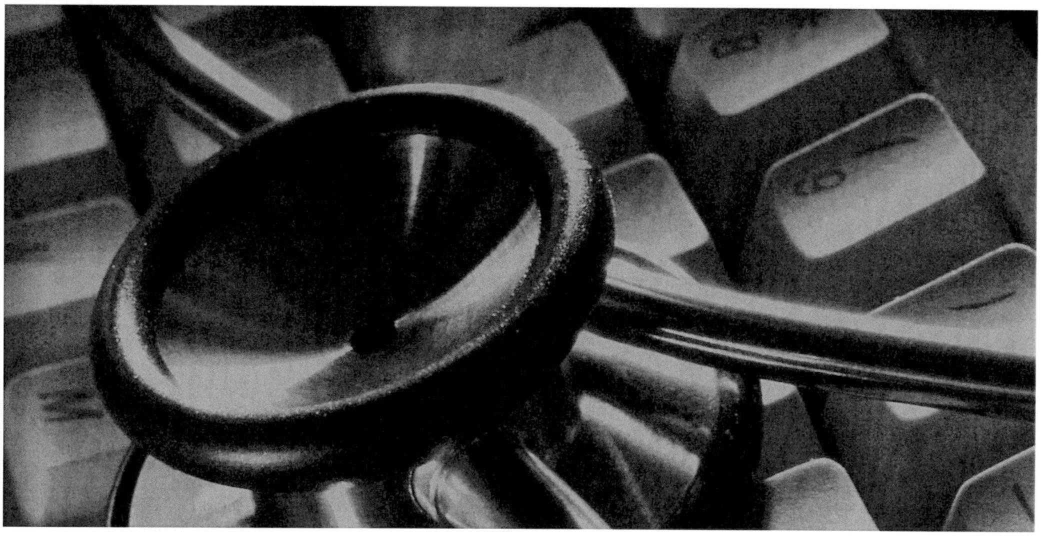

SECTION 5
Integrating Learners in Telehealth

Angelina Vascimini, Michelle B. McElhannon,* Andrew S. Tenpas, Eric Dietrich, and Holly Causey Canupp*

(*Equal effort as primary author)

CHAPTER 15
Review of Types of Learning Experiences

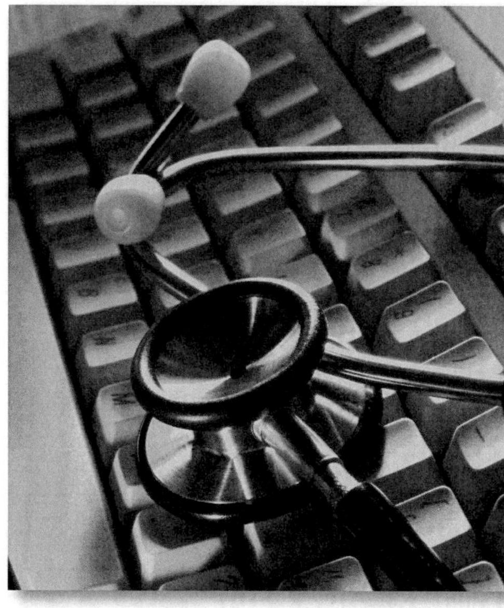

Just as face-to-face encounters can teach students and residents clinical and professional skills, incorporating learners into telehealth pharmacy practice can offer an experience that is unique, robust, and clinically challenging. Pharmacy-led telehealth patient encounters draw on different communication skill sets and allow students to engage in patient care remotely. Though challenging, adjusting or designing an experiential learning site to accommodate telehealth pharmacy practice models can be rewarding for preceptors, patients, and learners.

Training expectations and learning strategies for telehealth pharmacy practice rotations may differ based on whether the experience is an introductory pharmacy practice experience, an advanced pharmacy practice experience, or a postgraduate residency training experience.

INTRODUCTORY PHARMACY PRACTICE EXPERIENCES

Introductory pharmacy practice experiences (or IPPEs) generally consist of first-, second-, and even third-year pharmacy students seeking baseline exposure to general pharmacy practice. They may vary, however, depending on specific program duration and curriculum. Through short-term and long-term experiential opportunities, students can observe pharmacists and other members of the pharmacy team apply a wide variety of skills in different practice settings. IPPE rotations are structured to provide opportunities for career exploration across inpatient, outpatient, and specialized settings, as well as opportunities for student reflection, discussion, and professional development. Moreover, IPPE rotations allow student pharmacists to safely model techniques and practices under preceptor supervision. In 1997, the Accreditation Council for Pharmacy Education (ACPE) required experiential hours as part of a doctor of pharmacy (PharmD) degree. In this first reference, pharmacy students are generally required to complete at least 300 hours of IPPE experience divided between community and institutional practice settings.[1] However, due to some of the inherent ambiguity in ACPE standards, significant variation in IPPE rotational design has been noted between pharmacy programs. Although each pharmacy program and state may have its own IPPE requirements for successful graduation and licensure, the overarching structure is intended to be roughly similar across the country. This chapter is not intended to provide an in-depth review of IPPE requirements; the reader is encouraged to reference the individual requirements of their pharmacy program and state.

DOI 10.37573/9781585286928.015

In response to COVID-19 and its impact on didactic and experiential education opportunities, ACPE and the American College of Clinical Pharmacy (ACCP) released a joint statement to pharmacy programs across the country, declaring that "student opportunities using telehealth may count for ambulatory care or IPPE hours if they meet the competencies developed for your ambulatory care/IPPE rotations."[2] This signifies that educational organizations recognize that telehealth can serve an invaluable role in helping rotation sites meet curricular objectives and deadlines.[2] In addition, ACPE and ACCP do not give specific guidance on how to conduct telehealth rotations. Innovation is encouraged, as long as standards and curriculum objectives are met.[2]

ADVANCED PHARMACY PRACTICE EXPERIENCES

Conversely, advanced pharmacy practice experience (APPEs) feature student pharmacists prior to graduation, seeking more intensive and complex pharmacy practice opportunities. In general, rotations tend to be longer than those of IPPE students, and experiences tend to have elevated complexities that are more akin to what is seen in practice. Although student pharmacists still require supervision by a pharmacy preceptor, far greater autonomy is expected and given. Each program and state may have its own APPE requirements for graduation and licensure; interested readers are encouraged to reference the individual requirements of their pharmacy program and state. According to Danielson et al.,[3] the essential elements of core APPE experiences should include the following:

- Inpatient General Medicine and Ambulatory Care APPE rotations:
  - Pharmacist patient care
  - Communication and education
  - Interprofessional collaboration
  - Evidence-based medicine (EBM)
  - Practice-specific responsibilities (PSR)
- Community Pharmacy APPE rotations:
  - Pharmacist patient care
  - Communication and education
  - Population health
  - Dispensing system and safety management
  - Practice management

In a recent presentation, the executive director of ACPE wrote that while "the majority of APPE hours must involve direct patient-care . . . telehealth can be direct-patient care if designed appropriately." This again demonstrates that, with enough creativity and innovation, any APPE rotation can utilize telehealth to provide a challenging and personally rewarding experience for student pharmacists.[4]

POSTGRADUATE RESIDENCIES

Following graduation, many pharmacy students choose to complete postgraduate training. Residencies are traditionally classified as either postgraduate year 1 (PGY1) or postgraduate year 2 (PGY2), and residents can opt to pursue training in areas ranging from population-focused (e.g., pediatrics or geriatrics), disease-focused (e.g., oncology, cardiology, or others), or specialized settings (e.g., critical care, ambulatory care, pharmacogenomics, management). The American Society of Health-System Pharmacists (ASHP) maintains specific accreditation standards for both PGY1 and PGY2 residencies. Successful completion of an ASHP-accredited PGY1 program or a PGY1 program in candidacy status seeking accreditation is often required to progress to an ASHP-accredited

PGY2 program. In general, the ASHP-required competency areas and goals for PGY1 residencies are available at https:www.ashp.org.[5] While they will not be listed in full here, several observations can be made.

For one, there is significant overlap in several of the core competency areas and goals for residency training. While evaluation criteria are subject to change with time, a number of principles relating to patient care, education, leadership, and practice management are timeless and are not easily rooted out. It is important for preceptors, given the inherent ambiguity and subsequent variation found between IPPE, APPE, and resident rotations among programs, to identify and develop rotational experiences that draw on these core skill sets, especially when creating telehealth-based rotations.

Additionally, when reviewing the individual components of each competency area for both PGY1 and PGY2 residencies, two competencies have opportunities for telehealth: R1: Patient Care and E3: Initiating an Advanced Practice Area-Related Service. R1: Patient Care, for example, entails interacting with patients and caregivers, ensuring continuity of care between different settings, and collecting information on which to base safe and effective therapy.[5] Conversely, by designing, implementing, and assessing a new telehealth-based service (as outlined in E3), residents can develop the skill sets needed to fully utilize this treatment modality.

The core elements of each level of pharmacy learner experience are required to transition with the learning site as patient care pivots to pharmacy telehealth practice. Developing innovative learning opportunities and activities that continue to allow mastery of essential pharmacy skill sets will ensure successful telehealth pharmacy practice teaching and learning. Telehealth can be incorporated into each of the five pieces of the Joint Commission of Pharmacy Practitioners Pharmacists' Patient Care Process (**Figure 15.1**).[6] In the Practitioners Pharmacists' Patient Care Process, essential skills for pharmacy graduates and postgraduates are identified by preceptors to include areas of entrustability, including communication, teamwork, and professionalism.[7] Once essential skills have been identified, preceptors can follow the guidance from ACPE and ACCP to create innovative telehealth rotations that meet competencies and standards.

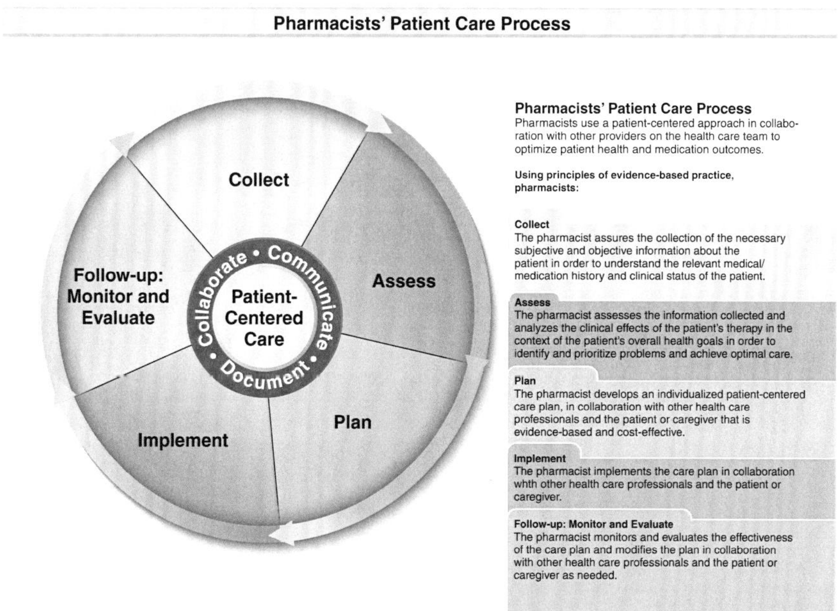

Figure 15.1. Pharmacists' Patient Care Process[7]

Source: https://jcpp.net/wp-content/uploads/2016/03/PatientCareProcess-with-supporting-organizations.pdf

Tool for Critical Skill Coverage in Pharmacy Telehealth Practice

Identified Elements of Essential Pharmacy Practice Skills for Pharmacy Graduates:
☐ Patient-Centered Care, Pharmacists' Patient Care Process (see Figure 15.1)
☐ Communication with patients, preceptors, and healthcare team
☐ Critical thinking
☐ Collaboration
☐ Vital signs and laboratory value evaluation and assessment
☐ Prescription evaluation
☐ Drug information
☐ Professionalism
☐ Cultural competence

REFERENCES

1. Accreditation Council for Pharmacy Education. Accreditation standards and key elements for the professional program in pharmacy leading to the doctor of pharmacy degree. **https://www.acpe-accredit.org/pdf/Standards2016FINAL.pdf**. Accessed May 5, 2021.
2. Accreditation Council for Pharmacy Education. Guidance memos from ACPE to schools. **https://www.acpe-accredit.org/wp-content/uploads/guidance-memos-from-ACPE-to-the-schools-consolidated-5-8-20.pdf**. Accessed May 5, 2021.
3. Danielson J, Besinque KH, Clarke C, et al. Essential elements for core required advanced pharmacy practice experiences. *Am J Pharm Educ*. 2019;83(4):6865. doi:10.5688/ajpe6865.
4. Accreditation Council for Pharmacy Education. ACPE update: Assuring quality in pharmacy education amid a pandemic. **https://www.acpe-accredit.org/pdf/ACPEUpdateASHPMCM2020updatedtableshandout.pdf**. Accessed May 5, 2021.
5. American Society of Health-System Pharmacists. Guidance document for the ASHP accreditation standard for postgraduate year one (PGY1) pharmacy residency programs. **https://www.ashp.org/-/media/assets/professional-development/residencies/docs/guidance-document-PGY1-standards.ashx?la=en&hash=20D275DC632B78E92626D7233DF52747279FE820**. Accessed May 5, 2021.
6. Joint Commission of Pharmacy Practitioners. Pharmacists' Patient Care Process. 2014. **https://jcpp.net/wp-content/uploads/2016/03/PatientCareProcess-with-supporting-organizations.pdf**. Accessed May 1, 2021.
7. Frenzel J, Eukel H, Neville M, et al. Essential skills for pharmacy graduates reported by advanced pharmacy practice experience preceptors. *Curr Pharm Teach Learn*. October 2015;700-704. doi: 10.1016/j.cptl.2015.06.005.

CHAPTER 16
Preparation for Telehealth Pharmacy Practice as a Learning Environment

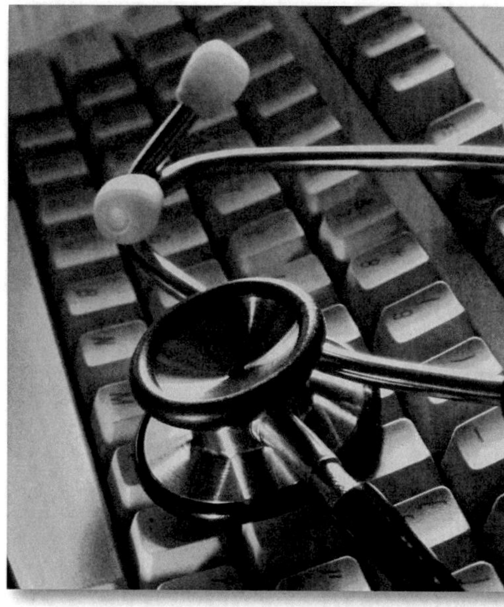

As telehealth pharmacy practice becomes more integrated into clinical care models, it is important to consider how this medium may impact pharmacy learning experiences. The rigor of the learning experience and the teaching of essential skill sets must be maintained in the telehealth practice model. This new care approach can allow for creative methods to learning, whether creating a new experience or adapting an existing one. Successful preparation of sites, preceptors, and learners is imperative for successful integration of learners into telehealth pharmacy practice models.

General steps to preparing telehealth pharmacy practice sites for learners include:

1. Site preparation
2. Patient care experience preparation
3. Evaluations preparation

PREPARING THE CLINICAL SITE FOR TELEHEALTH PHARMACY PRACTICE LEARNERS

Although site preparations will vary depending on the type of telehealth provided, evaluating the experiential learning environment and meeting site requirements for learner participation remains constant. A well-developed site integrates both the patient care environment and the environment in which teaching and learning occur[1] where the structure of the telehealth learning environment should enhance and complement the patient care environment (see **Figure 16.1**). When preparing different clinical and learning environments that will be provided via telehealth, initial evaluations should consider necessary resources. Resident and student preparation will differ. Residents have the ability to practice independently of their preceptor, as they are licensed pharmacists, and as such they do not require direct supervision. However, students will be licensed pharmacy interns, thus requiring additional space for preceptor oversight or direct supervision for certain activities (varying based on state pharmacy legislation). The physical space must be large enough to accommodate the number of pharmacy learners adherent to site and experience requirements for group interactions, preceptor oversight, distancing, and the like, while also offering private space as needed for HIPAA-compliant patient care, individual projects, and preceptor feedback. Access to the electronic health record and/or patient charts may require authorization for distance accessibility if the physical space onsite is inadequate and a remote location is needed. The site's technical support should be evaluated and a plan developed in anticipation of technical failures. In addition to computer access, a phone that allows three-way calling can be useful for preceptor use in modeling patient care and learner oversight, as well as enabling

DOI 10.37573/9781585286928.016

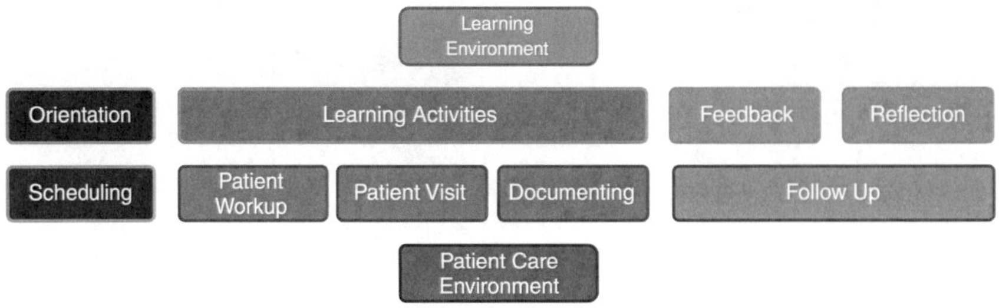

Figure 16.1. Integrating learners into the patient care environment

interpreter services. Learners will also benefit from access to drug information and primary literature resources either online or onsite.

Site-related learner requirements may come from the pharmacy program, institution, and state and/or local government, and will require the preceptor to navigate and resolve any conflicting or ambiguous requirements of the learner. Examples include clarifying any needed immunizations and testing (e.g., PPD, influenza, COVID-19), as well as defining the frequency of testing if the experience is ongoing or longitudinal. If learners are remote and interacting via distance experiential learning, the plan will need to consider how to obtain confidentiality agreements, background checks, drug testing, and any other requirements. In addition to site preferences, individual states likely differ in terms of required preceptor oversight and student supervision and may need clarification for telehealth purposes.

Beyond physical resources, it is important to ensure that the telehealth pharmacy practice experiences offer the same number and variety of patient encounters as a traditional face-to-face experience to ensure attainment of course goals and objectives. Sites that offer the addition of support staff to provide assistance with nonclinical activities such as scheduling, verifying patient eligibility, confirming patient accessibility to connective resources, and calling for appointment reminders can allow more time for clinical services and provide a more efficient teaching experience.[2,3]

Tool for Telehealth Pharmacy Practice Experiences

Site Preparation Checklist

1. SITE-SPECIFIC REQUIREMENTS	**4. INFORMATION**
☐ Immunization, physicals, background checks ☐ Confidentiality agreements, method to obtain agreements	☐ Drug information resources: availability and accessibility ☐ Primary literature resources: availability and accessibility
2. SPACE/PHYSICAL CAPACITY	**5. QUALITY EXPERIENCES**
☐ Group working space with appropriate distancing or ventilation ☐ Private space to conduct remote pharmacy visits ☐ Confidential patient space (if visit occurs from office setting)	☐ Site offers number and variety of patients with technology literacy/resources ☐ Site offers staff support to ensure quality time with patients and students
3. TECHNOLOGY	**6. STATE-SPECIFIC REQUIREMENTS**
☐ Electronic health record access (onsite and remote) ☐ Telephone access (remote routing) ☐ Technology support	☐ Preceptor oversight requirements ☐ Telehealth care is fully and legally compliant

Software Considerations for Pharmacy Telehealth Practice

As part of site preparation for clinical rotations that will be using telehealth as a care platform, significant thought should be given to selection of the software that will be used. Medical institutions and/or pharmacy programs may have specific software already selected. However, if the reader has the opportunity to select such software, ideal attributes include the following:

1. Health Insurance Portability and Accountability Act (HIPAA) compliant
2. Family Educational Rights and Privacy Act (FERPA) compliant
3. Cost effective
4. Ease of use
5. Video/telephone capabilities*
6. Screen-sharing capabilities*
7. Chat feature
8. Simultaneous multi-user capabilities*
9. Applicable to a variety of devices, including computers, smartphones, and tablets as well as operating systems (iOS, Android)

*Important consideration for learners

HIPAA compliance. The U.S. Department of Health and Human Services (HHS) stresses the importance of maintaining HIPAA when providing telehealth services. When selecting a telehealth software, HHS recommends choosing vendors that will enter into a HIPAA business-associated agreement.[4] As telehealth continues to grow and evolve, HIPAA-compliant software will be developed and updated. The *HIPAA Journal* is a useful resource when searching for the most up-to-date HIPAA-related information, and it provides a checklist for HIPAA compliance.[5]

FERPA compliance. The acting director of the Student Privacy Policy Office of the U.S. Department of Education recently provided guidance on FERPA and remote learning in a presentation titled "FERPA & Remote Learning During COVID-19." When addressing specific technology and FERPA, it stated that "FERPA is a privacy rule and does not include explicit information security standards,"[6] meaning that FERPA does not require any specific technology requirements. However, regardless of whether education is occurring live or remotely, FERPA needs to be maintained.

Cost effectiveness. When selecting telehealth software, the reader may consider the initial cost of the application, as well as additional costs associated with distributing to providers, pharmacists, residents, and students. It may also be worth verifying patient costs to access and utilization of software. Ideally, the selected software will be easily distributed to rotating learners and free for patients to use.

Ease of use. Selected software should be easy for providers, patients, residents, and students to use. In addition, if the software supplies training videos for its users, this may significantly increase the benefit users derive from it.

Video/telephone capabilities. Ideally, software will give users the capability of conducting patient encounters via video or telephone conferencing. Video and telephone capabilities are important for patient populations with barriers to either communication mechanism. Known barriers include minimal/no access to the Internet/video cameras, lack of proficiency in using technology, and patient preferences to avoid video communications. However, the nature of the visit may require video communication (e.g., evaluation of bruising from an anticoagulant, peripheral edema), and this should be considered when scheduling the visit with the patient and discussing the method of telehealth pharmacy practice care delivery.

Highlighting Essential Components of Telehealth Software for Learners

The development of communication skills is essential for learners. According to the Accreditation Council for Pharmacy Education, Standard 3.6 identifies communication as a key component for student learners.[7] In addition, communication is highlighted throughout PGY1 and PGY2 ASHP Accreditation Standards.[8-10] As new forms of communication continue to be developed, it will be important for learners to master technological forms of communication such as video and telephone.

Screen-sharing capabilities. In order for students and residents to counsel patients safely and effectively, telehealth software should have the ability to screen share. Screen sharing allows students or residents to effectively display information on their screen for the patient, and it also allows preceptors to model chart reviews. With this feature, it is easier to counsel patients. For example, when starting insulin, it is important to ensure that the patient has a good understanding of how to administer the medication. A student or resident could pull up a video of administration steps for insulin to share with the patient.

Screen-sharing capabilities give preceptors the ability to mirror on-the-spot teaching and topic discussions in a virtual environment. Some software has the ability to not only screen share but also mimic a whiteboard as an additional tool to assist comprehension for visual learners.

Chat feature. In the same way that screen sharing assists students and residents with counseling patients, a chat feature can be utilized for counseling. For example, students and residents can type out instructions that the patient can save for later reference. The chat feature can also be used to supply website links to the patient regarding other counseling points. A good example might be inclusion of a hyperlink to the plate method for patients with diabetes. If the platform allows for private chat, this feature could also be used during live educational sessions to coach the learner for specific tasks or areas to cover without having the observing preceptor interrupt.

Simultaneous multi-user capabilities. This function allows preceptors to accompany students or check in on residents during a patient visit, as well as allowing more than one person to complete the appointment. For example, when appointments are scheduled in advance and a specific learner is not assigned to the appointment, it is useful to have a versatile link that any student, resident, or pharmacist can access to complete the appointment. The link can also be used by preceptors to check in on learners.

The ability of preceptors to view learners in a virtual setting is important for both evaluation and feedback and ensures that the learner is appropriately communicating accurate information to the patient. In instances where learners encounter a problem and require assistance, the ability to have multiple users simultaneously engage in the visit may allow preceptors to step in and assist the learner and solve any issues that develop.

Applicability to a variety of devices. Patients will have different preferences for how to communicate with their healthcare team in terms of telehealth delivery route (phone vs. video) or device, which may include a computer, smartphone, or tablet. These devices may run different operating systems such as iOS or Android. The ideal program will not only be applicable to a variety of devices but also to operating systems to give patients and providers the ability to use their preferred device for the telehealth pharmacy practice visit.

Evaluating and Selecting Multimedia for Learning

Anstey and Watson recently released a *Rubric for E-Learning Tool Evaluation,* which may offer pharmacy educators and preceptors a way to assess the capabilities of different e-learning tools to meet the needs of pharmacy students.[11,12] This rubric may prove useful in evaluating various multimedia platforms as sites prepare for their students and residents.

Tool for Evaluating Multimedia Selection[11,12]

Category	Criteria
Functionality: Does the tool serve its intended purpose well?	**Scale** Can be scaled to accommodate any size class and allow creation of smaller subgroups
	Ease of Use Has a user-friendly interface, allowing students and preceptors to become easily proficient
	Tech Support / Availability of Help Campus-based technical support or documentation is easily accessible, robust support platform for troubleshooting
	Hypermediality Allows user to communicate via different channels (audio, visual, textual); allows flexible/adaptive engagement with material
Accessibility: Does it support multiple learning approaches and engagement for all students?	**Accessibility Standards** Does it, at a minimum, adhere to mandated requirements for accessibility?
	User-Focused Participation Addresses the needs of different users with different literacies and capabilities
	Required Equipment Use of tool does not require equipment beyond normal capabilities of educators, preceptors, or students
	Cost of Use All aspects of tool can be used free of charge or at minimal cost
Technical: Does the technology have integral Internet access, software, hardware, and computer availability?	**Integration/Embedding within Learning Management System (LMS)** Can the tool be embedded into a LMS (.html), yet retain full functionality?
	Desktop/Laptop Operating Systems Can be utilized with any standard, up-to-date operating system
	Browser Can be utilized with any standard, up-to-date browser
	Additional Downloads Students or users do not need to download any additional software or extensions
Mobile Design: Can it deliver content using current and expanding mobile technology?	**Access** Can be downloaded as either an app or mobile browser; takes into account use of smaller-sized screen
	Functionality Little or no difference between mobile and desktop version
	Offline Access Offers offline mode, including continued access to core features/functions

(Continued)

Tool for Evaluating Multimedia Selection (*Continued*)

Category	Criteria
Privacy, Data Protection, and Rights: Does it adequately protect personal information and intellectual property?	**Sign Up / Sign In** Use of tool does not require external account or additional login
	Data Privacy and Ownership User can keep data private and decide if or how data are shared
	Archiving, Saving, and Exporting Data Can archive, save, import, and export content or data as needed
Social Presence: Does it allow participants to project their personal characteristics into the community, creating a safe, trusting environment for collaboration and teamwork?	**Collaboration** Able to support a community of users through synchronous and asynchronous opportunities
	User Accountability Has technical solutions to hold users accountable for their actions
	Diffusion Tool is widely known and popular; likely, nearly everyone has basic technical competence to use it
Teaching Presence: Does it enable instructors to establish and maintain their teaching presence through facilitation, customization, and feedback?	**Facilitation** Easy-to-use features allowing instructors/preceptors to actively engage, monitor, and provide feedback to students
	Customization Adaptable to the learning environment, easily customized to fit different contexts and learning outcomes
	Learning Analytics Instructors/preceptors can monitor student performance via a variety of measures and provide feedback via user-friendly dashboard
Cognitive Presence: Does it support students' cognitive engagement in learning tasks?	**Enhancement of Cognitive Tasks** Enhances engagement in tasks once thought overly complex or inconceivable via other means
	Higher-Order Thinking Allows users to exercise higher-order thinking skills
	Metacognitive Engagement Learners can regularly receive formative feedback on learning (track performance, monitor improvement, regularly test knowledge)

FURTHER PREPARING THE SITE: OBTAINING NECESSARY PERMISSIONS

Clinical Care: Obtaining Consents

Telehealth visits being conducted remotely require patient consent for insurance reimbursement. Additionally, it may be prudent to obtain patient consent if multiple parties participate in the visit such as students, residents, the primary clinical pharmacist, physicians, and nurses. Based on the nature of the visit and/or the patient's personal preferences, the patient may wish to limit the number of people involved in the visit, including those passively observing, making it important to address this issue at the very start of the visit. Outlining who will be conducting which element(s) of the visit establishes transparency with the patient and provides an opportunity to express patient preferences or concerns. In addition, by using remote means to complete the appointment, patients may be more willing to have observers as physical space limitations have been eliminated.

Methods to Communicate with Patients before, during, and after Telehealth Visits

Depending on the delivery mechanism of the telehealth pharmacy practice visit (telephone vs. video), patient-specific information may have to be delivered to the patient. For example, a link for a video visit will be patient-, date-, and time-specific, and may also need to be specific for the pharmacist or learner completing the telehealth pharmacy practice visit (see the earlier section in this chapter titled Software Considerations for Pharmacy Telehealth Practice). The clinic will have to determine how to communicate this information to the patient. Based on the type of visit and resources available, information may be transmitted via secure messaging within the electronic health record (EHR), directly emailing the patient, mailing information through traditional mail, or providing the information to the patient over the phone prior to the visit. The patient's preferred mechanism of communication should be determined, although the method of communication may depend largely on the route of telehealth delivery. Furthermore, if email is the preferred route, the clinic should consider who will be sending the patient the message, as it may be through an email of the clinic staff or pharmacist who may not wish to provide a personal email to patients. Use of institutional email sent to outside addresses may also compromise security. It is reasonable to consider including additional information in the email message concerning simple steps on how to use the telehealth software, to reply to that email for technical help, to ask clinical questions, or to provide emergency issues and specific instructions regarding whom the patient should contact if questions arise.

Lastly, preceptors will have to determine who will send information to the patient. Based on the type of information, the sender may include clinic staff (most likely for logistical information related to the visit, who to contact for technical support, etc.), the pharmacist preceptor, or the learner. If the learner is to be responsible for sending information, they should not have to use their personal, school, or residency email address to communicate with the patient. Ideally, the electronic medical record would be used to send information to the patient, with the additional advantage of being available to other members of the healthcare team for continuity. The preceptor should be able to review the information first for accuracy and completeness before it is sent to the patient. The preceptor may also have to implement a process to educate learners on the appropriate strategies to communicate information and appropriate verbiage to utilize, and also to vet the learner's ability to communicate via this mechanism prior to allowing the learner to send information to the patient. However, this will be highly dependent on the learner (IPPE, APPE, resident) and practice setting, and the process will have to be adjusted accordingly. The preceptor may consider separate training in this area, developing a "Best Practices Guide" or having patient cases to work through ahead of time to provide practice opportunities for the learners and clarifying questions. This practice approach will also allow the preceptor to gauge learner skillset, identify areas that require additional coaching, and provide feedback.

Defining Plans for Research or Quality Assessment Projects Regarding Learner Involvement in Pharmacy Telehealth Practice

Given the novelty of providing medication management services via telehealth, as well as creating, re-designing, and/or implementing telehealth-based learning experiences for a variety of learners, pharmacists may perform practice-based research, quality improvement projects, or education-based research evaluating the new or different models they are working within.[13] Student learners may be interested in completing research projects, while residents will likely be required to complete a project. While the novelty of delivering healthcare and education via telehealth provides unique opportunities for research, it also introduces additional challenges that must be identified and addressed.

Based on the nature of a clinical project, the local Institutional Review Board (IRB) may require informed consent from the patient, depending on the focus of the research. It is important for the pharmacist to consult with their local IRB to determine whether telehealth-focused projects require IRB approval or if approval can be granted as a continuous quality improvement (CQI) project. These determinations would then guide the pharmacist with respect to what kind of patient consent, if any, would be required to collect and share data from these visits. If the IRB requires informed consent, it is important to ensure that the personnel obtaining informed consent are listed as researchers on the project. Students and/or residents rotating through the practice site on a short-term basis may not be listed on the project and therefore should not be the ones obtaining informed consent from the patient for the research-related aspects of the visit.

For education-based projects, informed consent may be required from the learners who will be the study participants. Given that students may be considered a vulnerable population, special attention will have to be given to the IRB and consenting process. Furthermore, if the nature of the research is behavioral or survey-based, the local IRB may have different and/or additional requirements than are required for traditional clinical projects. If the project is describing changes made to an experience or discussing high-level considerations for restructuring or delivering learning experiences through telehealth, it may not require formal IRB approval, but it may be prudent to check with the local IRB before starting the project.[14]

QUALITY AND OUTCOME ASSESSMENTS FOR LEARNERS ENGAGED IN PHARMACY TELEHEALTH PRACTICE

Developing a quality assessment program is instrumental in ensuring that the experience is delivering both high-quality patient care and student/resident learning opportunities. Hard metrics used to assess the patient care environment, such as number of patients seen and number of clinical interventions, can also be used to evaluate the quality and variety of the student/resident learning environment and see that learners are provided an appropriate number of opportunities to make clinical interventions.

In addition to utilizing student site evaluations after the experience, assessment of qualitative measures throughout the experience is important. Input from staff, clinicians, students, and patients should be solicited to track satisfaction metrics on both the patient and student/resident experiences. Possible survey questions could include the following:

- How has the telehealth pharmacy practice experience impacted student/resident satisfaction?
- How has student/resident integration impacted patient satisfaction?
- How has student/resident integration affected provider satisfaction?
- How has student/resident integration influenced patient outcomes?

Workflow quality assessments should also be included, noting time of student engagement at each step, as well as technology benefits and limitations. Preceptors should look for opportunities to restructure and improve the processes and learning experiences if problems are identified. Given the novelty of providing both patient care and education functions in a telehealth environment, it is expected that adjustments will be required. In addition, routine assessment of the service, both clinically and from an educational perspective, will be needed to ensure changes are made in a timely manner.

As society demands improved teaching and awareness of cultural competency, other areas for focused consideration include tracking for diversity of patient encounters during the telehealth platforms, social determinants that create barriers for telehealth use, or disabilities that may influence care quality if not considered. Learners need to have skills ranging across various social determinants of health. Thus, it is important to comprehensively introduce students to a wide diversity of patients so that they may be exposed to varied approaches necessary to improve the patient care outcome. Another often overlooked consideration is the healthcare worker's implicit bias, which may offer interesting discussions with learners trying to implement care with telehealth modalities.[15]

PREPARING THE LEARNING EXPERIENCE TO HIGHLIGHT PHARMACY TELEHEALTH PRACTICES

In traditional experiential teaching, consistency and standardization are essential for effective teaching, and the same remains true for integrating students and residents into a telehealth pharmacy practice experience.[16] To provide a learning environment that supplements the clinical environment, the preceptor should be prepared to evaluate the learning objectives, structure and workflow of the experience, preceptor and learner training, the quality of patient encounters, and clinical and educational outcomes.

Establishing Goals and Objectives

Preparation for the telehealth pharmacy practice experience starts with determining how goals and objectives will be practiced and assessed for student/resident ambulatory learning. Experiential requirements may need to be adjusted to account for the delivery of services via telehealth, though the extent may depend on a variety of factors including:

- The route(s) of delivery of telehealth pharmacy practice services
- The proportion of clinical services provided in-person versus telehealth
- The location of the learner (clinic site only, home only, or a hybrid)
- Scope and types of services offered including, but not limited to, medication management, medication reconciliation, patient counseling and education, or vaccine administration
- Opportunities (or lack thereof) for collaboration with other healthcare providers
- Opportunities (or lack thereof) for physical assessment skills such as blood pressure, point-of-care blood glucose, HbA1c, or INR testing, foot exams
- Opportunities for documentation regarding patient interactions and care plan development

If objectives are not met or are not adequately evaluated, alternative options should be explored. While simply delaying assessment of these skills until a later rotation may seem reasonable, the schedule of the learner and the number and type of rotations remaining may not allow for assessment of certain skills.

If certain objectives cannot be met during the course of the rotation due to lack of access to direct patient care or lack of remote access to the electronic health record, creativity in achieving the objectives is required. Identified gaps in the experience can be supplemented with self-directed learning such as journal clubs, topic discussions, drug information questions, and case studies. Asking the residents or students to present the next clinical step after independently researching the topic can challenge learners efficiently and complement the telehealth encounter.[17]

Tool for Meeting Objectives in the Virtual Environment[13,19,20]

Supplementary Asynchronous Ambulatory Care Activities in the Telehealth Pharmacy Experience
☐ Medication therapy management (MTM) reviews
☐ Prior authorization processing
☐ Medication assistance program enrollment coordination
☐ Drug information handout creation
☐ Drug information questions
☐ Writing activities (case reports, review articles, student reflections, etc.)
☐ Data analysis
☐ Quality assurance
☐ Educational session (in-services, grand rounds, etc.)

In cases where the assessment of certain objectives is not feasible (e.g., vaccine administration, physical assessment skills) due to services being provided exclusively via telehealth, the preceptor may have to evaluate these skills outside of a patient care episode. It may be possible for certain learners to demonstrate some of these skills on a consenting person living in their household/co-learner on the same rotation while the preceptor observes remotely in real time or a recording of the learner performing the assessment skills. Some skills, such as vaccine administration, may necessitate assessment through a discussion with the learner who would verbally walk through the required elements or through a written assessment created by the preceptor to evaluate specific techniques and skills. While these routes of assessment are not preferred to assessment completed on a live patient, they may be required if in-person clinical services cannot be provided. Alternative options may also include instructing the learner to develop their own training video and record themselves performing the steps in a simulation-type setting with the use of training aids or on another student.

Outlining the Workflow for Learning Engagement in Pharmacy Telehealth Practice

After determining the goals and objectives of the experience, preceptors should develop a workflow plan for learner integration into telehealth pharmacy practice visits that take into account both patient care and student learning or teaching environment. Successful integration of students into the telehealth process is a team effort, and engagement of clinic staff, clinicians, and IT personnel is necessary to provide input on workflow design and identify areas in the patient care environment where the student experience will fit. Different models will need to be created for students and residents, assuming the resident acquires licensure in the state. While oversight is still necessary, the intensity is different than with a student learner.

- Opportunity #1: The pharmacy clinician schedules patients rather than having support staff, leaving less time for student interaction.
- Solution #1: If support staff are not available, students can be involved in patient scheduling and preparation, particularly if clinical baseline questions are incorporated at this stage.
- Opportunity #2: Patients are unfamiliar with telehealth procedures, which makes the experience less efficient.
- Solution #2: Patients may need an orientation to the telehealth procedure and tips to facilitate the visit. The student can be included in assessing patients' health literacy and barriers to care and can be asked to reflect on the early contact points of the encounter.

Establishing a Technology Orientation Process for Learners

Many student/resident experiences are blocked rather than longitudinal. Establish a plan to train preceptors, students, and residents on the telehealth platform that will be used. In addition to training information concerning the platform, incorporation of training specific to telehealth communication strategies is essential. Training resources and expectations for self-study should be communicated to learners before the experience in addition to onsite training and reinforcement.

Tools for Establishing a Technology Orientation Process

Training Tips

- ☐ Check with vendor about the availability of training support resources.
- ☐ Develop or obtain from your vendor written and/or training materials that learners and preceptors can use.
- ☐ Develop or obtain from your vendor patient educational materials that learners can be taught to use to support different patient learning styles.
- ☐ Provide resources ahead of the rotation for prep work and training.
- ☐ Set clear expectations of learners' self-directed learning and timeframe to complete.
- ☐ Schedule time for preceptor-directed learner training and reinforcement.

CONDUCTING EVALUATIONS DURING OR VIA TELEHEALTH

Telehealth integration into learning models highlights the need for optimized evaluation. Evaluations can be broken into two major types: formative and formal.

Formative Evaluations

Remote rotations may offer fewer in-person interactions, and it may become difficult for preceptors to give on-the-spot, formative feedback to learners. This problem can be alleviated by setting up "pulse checks" with learners. Pulse checks can be defined as a quick tool for formative feedback. Preceptors may set up pulse checks on a weekly or daily basis, and they consist of on-the-spot feedback dependent on the learners' progress at that time. The goal of pulse checks is similar to that of in-person or on-sight rotations. However, with remote rotations, it may be more important to have frequent check-ins with learners to maintain the flow of communication and preceptor–learner relationships. "Remote Coffee Hour" and "Remote Lunch Breaks," which encourage providing feedback during an informal virtual social setting, have been utilized in the professional arena and can be useful to help coworkers feel less isolated when working from remote locations.[20] This concept can be applied to learners on remote rotations. These daily or weekly pulse checks can have a designated time determined at the start of the rotation and can be incorporated during breaks or mealtimes. Formative evaluations can also be spur-of-the-moment efforts to give the learner feedback in real time. In some cases, preceptors may find it is important to have both designated times set aside as well as opportunities for feedback in real time.

Tool for Pulse Checks

Pulse checks should encompass the following:

- ☐ Feedback on learner's performance from a patient care and professionalism standpoint
- ☐ Feedback from learners to address concerns they may have, to discuss their learning experience so far, and to ensure the learner feels supported by the preceptor
- ☐ Mental health check-ins to discuss feelings of inclusivity versus isolation due to less in-person interaction
- ☐ Knowledge checks to ensure learners' progression should be expected throughout the rotation

Formal Evaluations

Formal evaluation may be less affected by remote learning environments than formative evaluations. Formal evaluation is data-driven, occurs after a particular learning cycle has ended, compares one student to expected outcome threshold for performance (e.g., exam scores), and may not be immediately actionable. Examples of such evaluations include writing assignments and formal exams.[21]

It is still imperative for preceptors to have clear-cut expectations and objectives for IPPE and APPE students and residents when conducting formal evaluations. A recent work by Boyle and colleagues[22] examined student perceptions of IPPE rotations. Overall, students had less favorable expectations of their preceptors to develop site-specific goals and objectives, and they were less confident in creating and sharing their own personal and professional goals with those preceptors following their IPPEs.[22] To provide greater focus on the development of pharmacy curricula and student rotational experiences, the Center for the Advancement of Pharmacy Education (CAPE)[23] developed specific educational outcomes intended to highlight the unique role pharmacists played on the healthcare team and expand the clinical roles and responsibilities of future pharmacists. The reader is encouraged to access a complete listing of outcomes on the AACP website. Comprising 4 domains and 15 subdomains, many of the 2013 CAPE Educational Outcomes link directly to telehealth. Two examples are immediately apparent. First, the domain "Essentials for Practice and Care" discusses collecting and interpreting evidence, formulating assessments, and monitoring and adjusting plans. Second, the domain "Approach to Patient Care" highlights recognizing social determinants of health (like economic stability and access to certain technologies) to eliminate disparities in patient access to care. All of these skills can be drawn upon in a telehealth environment and should be encouraged by preceptors and residency directors.[23]

The American Association of Colleges of Pharmacy (AACP) designed Entrustable Professional Activities (or EPAs), which are essential activities or tasks that all new pharmacy graduates—whether entering the workforce or pursuing residency training—must be able to perform without supervision. AACP suggests that graduates should be "independently executable, observable, and measurable in their process and outcome." The following EPAs serve as bare minimum competencies for newly minted pharmacists.[24] The reader is encouraged, once again, to access a more comprehensive listing of EPAs on the AACP website. Of the 15 listed activities, at least one-third tie directly to telehealth and its opportunities for patient care, notably:

- Collect information to identify a patient's medication-related problems and health-related needs.
- Analyze information to determine the effects of medication therapy, identify medication-related problems, and prioritize health-related needs.
- Follow up and monitor a care plan.
- Identify patients at risk for prevalent diseases in a population.
- Educate patients and professional colleagues regarding the appropriate use of medications.

Since such a high level of importance is placed on these activities in real-life practice—and they are witnessed in nearly every sector of pharmacy practice—it is essential that preceptors and other evaluators instill and cultivate these skill sets within their students' pharmacists. While on rotation, telehealth pharmacy practice encounters could help students to further develop their ability to quickly assess a patient and their individualized needs, educate that patient about their therapy and potential side effects, and then successfully follow that patient longitudinally. No matter where a student pharmacist eventually practices, these foundational principles are essential.

When rotations are transitioned to remote learning settings, formal evaluation may not be directly impacted by this transition. However, to ensure all accreditation standards and residency standards are met, additional emphasis may be placed on key pieces of formal evaluations.

Formal elements of evaluation for rotational students:

1. Disease state knowledge
2. Drug therapy evaluations and development
3. Monitoring for end points
4. Patient case presentations*
5. Patient interviews*
6. Patient education/counseling*

7. Drug information
8. Formal oral presentations*
9. Formal written presentations*
10. Professional team interaction*
11. Professionalism/motivation
12. Culture sensitivity

*Special consideration for telehealth rotations

Formal elements of evaluations for residents:

- Patient care*
- Advancing practice and improving patient care*
- Leadership and management
- Teaching, education, and dissemination of knowledge*

*Special consideration for telehealth rotations

Special consideration may be placed on certain aspects of formal evaluations. When learners are completing patient interactions via telehealth, unforeseen challenges may be encountered when presenting patients to preceptors, interviewing patients, and providing education or counseling to patients. While the specific criteria used to evaluate learners will not change, as quality patient care still needs to occur regardless of the setting, the means to meet these standards have changed and may require more coaching from preceptors. While remote rotations and experiences will provide unique challenges, formal evaluations remain important benchmarks for learners as well as preceptors and should cover all aspects of the learning experience.

PREPARING THE LEARNER FOR PHARMACY TELEHEALTH PRACTICE

To provide the foundation for a successful experience whether remotely or in person, it is ideal to create a well-organized orientation that occurs at the beginning of each learning experience. While a well-structured orientation will likely create an increased workload upfront, it will also ensure a smoother experience for the learner during the rotation.

Part of the orientation may include a checklist for essential tools required of the learner for the experience.

Tool for Essential Resources Required for Learner Experience

Sample Resource Checklist
☐ Internet
☐ Computer/hardware (i.e., widescreen monitor, working computer, quality headphones/microphones)
☐ Quiet work area that ensures clinical activities (i.e., phone calls) can be completed in private
☐ Resources for drug information requests
☐ Capability for contacting patients via phone (i.e., HIPAA-compliant phone app)
☐ Resources for communicating with preceptor real-time during clinical activities

Once orientation is under way, preceptors must embrace innovation and creativity to optimize the learning experience, as this can make for a better experience for both the learner and the preceptor. Early in the experience, topic discussions could be batched remotely to gauge the learner's baseline knowledge and to prepare the learner for patients seen either in person or as telehealth pharmacy practice. Nondirect patient care activities can occur via a remote platform without jeopardizing the learning experience.[13,25] For instance, with learning experiences in which learners are onsite for some of the time and remote for the remainder of the time, a half-day per week may be devoted to completing topic discussions and journal clubs via a remote platform.

Discussion of expectations and scheduled check-ins with learners are vital for remote-based experiences. Learners may feel apprehensive that the experience may not be able to provide them with direct patient care opportunities (especially those interested in ambulatory care) or that they will not have enough opportunity to develop crucial relationships with preceptors that may benefit them as future career opportunities arise.[26] In addition, anecdotal evidence suggests that learning experiences, which are 100% remote or hybridized, can feel isolating. While preceptors are in charge of precepting the clinical experience, they are also responsible for fostering both personal and professional growth during the rotation. The key to success for such growth is to promote personal resilience and care for the learner's well-being. The following may be considered in order to promote resilience and well-being in our learners during times of change:

- Upfront and clear expectations
- Assurance that learning objectives will be met regardless of direct patient care opportunities
- Regular check-ins with the learner to ensure progression on rotation activities
- Regular check-ins with learners to gauge how things are going personally
- Emergency and backup contact information so that the preceptor is readily accessible

WORKING THROUGH BARRIERS WHILE PREPARING A TELEHEALTH PHARMACY PRACTICE LEARNING EXPERIENCE

Barrier 1: Transition to Remote-Based Learning Environments (Students and Residents)

- The majority of teaching prior to rotations happens live within the classroom setting for students and within the clinical setting for residents. The majority of students and residents have had minimal learning experiences/encounters remotely. Also, students and residents are commonly prepared to complete rotations in person with preceptors and patients. These common practices do not prepare students for the transition to remote patient care experiences.

Solution 1: Incorporate Brief Training in Student and Resident Orientation to a Clinical Experience

- Orientation for students and residents typically consists of familiarizing learners with the physical practice site, workflow, and expectations/responsibilities. For remote rotations, the focus of orientation may shift. Instead of familiarizing learners with the physical practice site, preceptors can spend time reviewing how to use the telehealth software and the electronic health record. This can be done with the preceptor or on the learners' own time with training videos or modules provided by the telehealth software and/or the institution. Orientation to workflow and setting expectations/responsibilities will also shift to focus on remote interactions. Differences will occur in how and when learners will need to report to preceptors, whether in reference to patients, projects, questions, and so on. In addition, clearly defined expectations will need to be set, with emphasis on telehealth/remote encounters.

Barrier 2: Possible Reduction to Patient Access/Patient Encounters

- Because of the inherent challenges of telehealth related to technological literacy and to limited access to technology/Internet, remote rotations may have a smaller number of available patients to be seen during a rotation dependent on population.

Solution 2: Alternative Projects Focused on Clinical Knowledge and Patient Care

- According to Standard 13 of the Accreditation Council for Pharmacy Education, APPE students are not required to see a certain number of patients; however, they "should be exposed to a minimum of 160 hours in each required APPE area."[7] This concept holds true for residents as well. According to ASHP Duty Hour Requirements, pharmacy residents must complete a specific number of hours on each rotation.[27] With a decrease in patient touch points, preceptors will need to have prepared projects/assessments to replace the time learners would usually spend with patients. These projects/assessments should be focused on clinical knowledge or patient care, providing the learners with experiences analogous to patient care.
    - Project/Assessment Examples
        - Patient Case Development: Have learners create a patient case focusing on a specific disease state. Along with this case, have learners develop questions to go along with it. Learners will have to review the disease state in depth in order to create a complex case with thought-provoking questions.
        - Note Template Development: Have learners create a note template they would want to use to help guide themselves through patient interviews. This gives learners the opportunity to work through what information is important to gather on a subjective level and what information is needed to make clinical decisions. Further, it creates opportunities to have learners justify the importance and relevance of the interview questions to encourage a deeper understanding behind the structure and focus of an interview for a particular disease state.

Barrier 3: Patient Resistance to Telehealth Pharmacy Practice Appointment Types Coupled with Learners Providing Care

- In some instances, patients may express concern about the accuracy or efficacy of completing an appointment over telehealth. This worry may be amplified when a learner is completing the encounter, regardless of preceptor presence.

Solution 3: Empowering Learners to Explain the Details of Telehealth

- Patient resistance in this setting gives learners the opportunity to flex their communication skills. Throughout the rotation, learners will have the opportunity to observe their preceptors in order to see how to best alleviate a patient's fear. Preceptors can empower learners to explain what telehealth pharmacy practice is, what it will look like for the patient over the next several months, and what to expect from healthcare professionals. It will be important for preceptors to prepare learners for these conversations with patients, and opportunities to practice via role-playing scenarios may be necessary prior to learners engaging in conversations with patients. This is a vitally important skill for residents as they will be evaluating patients more autonomously as opposed to the supervised student interactions.

Barrier 4: Time Management

- Given the increased utilization of web-based platforms for telehealth, time spent on such applications as well as integrating other essential activities may be increased when compared to 100% face-to-face activities. Therefore, it might prove difficult to find enough time to complete the required patient care activities in addition to these other essential activities in remote learning environments.

Solution 4: Set Priorities and Remember Boundaries

- Integrate learners into practice early on to help with both clinical and nonclinical activities.
- See workflow incorporation suggestions under Outlining the Workflow for Learning Engagement in Pharmacy Telehealth Practice.
    - Evaluate points in the workflow where students can be integrated and design learning activities to complement the work function. Example: Learners can participate in scheduling, but add a clinical component such as a health literacy assessment that the learner can provide and reflect upon.

Barrier 5: Communication

- Learners should be prepped on best practices related to communicating via video or telephonic routes, as most didactic teaching is focused on in-person communication where body language and other nonverbal cues are able to be ascertained and communicated. However, some of these cues may not be received at all, such as when communicating exclusively over the phone, or they may be reduced when using video mechanisms of communication. The importance of speaking slowly and clearly should be emphasized, but learners should also be prepared to pause the conversation frequently to ensure the patient is appropriately following along, has understood what has been communicated, and has no additional questions. Utilization of the "teach back" method following counseling will likely be prudent to ensure the information conveyed by the learner was accurately received and internalized by the patient. If possible, it may also be important to send written instructions to the patient following the visit to ensure pertinent information is available to the patient after the visit has concluded.

Solution 5: Additional Practice with the Preceptor or Other Learners Will Likely Be Needed Prior to the Learner Completing Direct Patient Care Activities

- Ideally, these practice sessions should occur via the same delivery mechanism of the planned patient care services (telephonic, video) in order to more accurately simulate the expected environment in which the care will be provided.

REFERENCES

1. Fitzsimmon DS, Colbert J Jr, Hendley RT, et al. Preceptor-student relationship. In: Cuellar LM, Ginsburg DB (eds). *Preceptor's Handbook for Pharmacists*, 2nd ed.;2009:56-58. American Society of Health-System Pharmacists.
2. Schultz KW, Kirby J, Delva D, et al. Medical students' and residents' preferred site characteristics and preceptor behaviors for learning in the ambulatory setting: A cross-sectional survey. *BMC Med Educ*. August 6, 2004;4:12. doi: 10.1186/1472-6920-4-12.
3. Jaberizadeh L, Peterson J, Thrall S. Improving efficiency through workflow optimization in a pharmacist-run diabetes clinic. *Am J Health-Syst Pharm*. 2020;77(19):1606-1611. doi: 10.1093/ajhp/zxaa193.
4. FAQs on Telehealth and HIPAA during the COVID-19 Nationwide Public Health Emergency. U.S. Department of Health and Human Services Office for Civil Rights. October 2, 2020. **www.hhs.gov/sites/default/files/telehealth-faqs-508.pdf**. Accessed May 2, 2021.
5. "About HIPAA Journal." *HIPAA J*. November 20, 2020. **www.hipaajournal.com/hipaa-journal**. Accessed May 5, 2021.
6. Surprenant KS. "FERPA and Virtual Learning during COVID-19." Protecting Student Privacy.student privacy.ed.gov/training/ferpa-and-remote-learning-during-covid-19-webinar-recording. Accessed May 18, 2021.
7. "Accreditation Standards and Key Elements for the Professional Program in Pharmacy Leading to the Doctor of Pharmacy Degree." Accreditation Council for Pharmacy Education, 2015. **https://www.acpe-accredit.org/pdf/Standards2016FINAL.pdf**. Accessed May 18, 2021.
8. American Society of Health-System Pharmacists. Guidance document for the ASHP accreditation standard for postgraduate year one (PGY1) community-based pharmacy residency programs. **https://www.ashp.org/-/media/assets/professional-development/residencies/docs/guidance-document-PGY1-standards.ashx**. Accessed May 18, 2021.
9. American Society of Health-System Pharmacists. Guidance document for the ASHP accreditation standard for postgraduate year one (PGY1) pharmacy residency programs. **https://www.ashp.org/-/media/assets/professional-development/residencies/docs/guidance-document-PGY1-standards.ashx?la=en&hash=20D275DC632B78E92626D7233DF52747279FE820**. Accessed May 18, 2021.
10. American Society of Health-System Pharmacists. Guidance document for the ASHP accreditation standard for postgraduate year two (PGY2) pharmacy residency programs. **https://www.ashp.org/-/media/assets/professional-development/residencies/docs/pgy2-guidance-document.ashx?la=en&hash=47DDF4A2061DA39902C16622FB0EE7209BB**. Accessed May 18, 2021.
11. Anstey L, Watson G. A rubric for evaluating e-learning tools in higher education. **https://er.educause.edu/articles/2018/9/a-rubric-for-evaluating-e-learning-tools-in-higher-education**. Accessed May 18, 2021.
12. Anstey L, Watson G. Rubric for eLearning tool evaluation. **https://teaching.uwo.ca/pdf/elearning/Rubric-for-eLearning-Tool-Evaluation.pdf**. Accessed May 18, 2021.
13. Anderson S, Bianco J, DeRemer CE. Adapting ambulatory care learning environments in response to the COVID-19 pandemic. *Am J Health Syst Pharm.* 2021:78(6):467-471. **https://doi.org/10.1093/ajhp/zxab016**.
14. Moreau C, Maravent S, Hale GM, Joseph T. Strategies for managing pharmacy experiential education during COVID-19. *J Pharm Pract.* 2021;34(1):7-10. doi:10.1177/0897190020977730.
15. Avant ND, Gillespie GL. Pushing for health equity through structural competency and implicit bias education: A qualitative evaluation of a racial/ethnic health disparities elective course for pharmacy learners. *Curr Pharm Teach Learn*. April 2019;11(4):382-393. doi: 10.1016/j.cptl.2019.01.013.
16. Krause JE. Preceptor's handbook for pharmacists. *Am J Pharm Educ*. 2010;74(2):33 b.
17. Jeon M, Took RL, Gattas NM. Addressing challenges to precepting advanced pharmacy practice experience students in the community setting. *Curr Pharm Teach Learn*. 2020;12(7):872-877. doi: 10.1016/j.cptl.2020.02.005.
18. Elson E, Oermann C, Duehlmeyer S, Bledsoe S. Use of telemedicine to provide clinical pharmacy services during the SARS-CoV-2 pandemic. *Am J Health Syst Pharm.* 2020;77(13):1005–1006. **https://doi.org/10.1093/ajhp/zxaa112**.
19. Persky, A. Fuller KA, Jarstfer M, et al. Maintaining core values in postgraduate programs during the COVID-19 pandemic. *Am J Pharm Educ.* 2020;84(6). doi:10.5688/ajpe8158.

20. Murphy M. These two weird techniques will keep you connected to your team during isolation. *Forbes Magazine*. March 26, 2020. **www.forbes.com/sites/markmurphy/2020/03/26/these-two-weird-techniques-will-keep-you-connected-to-your-team-during-isolation/?sh=7980d9f1398e**. Accessed May 18, 2021.
21. Wright JL. Assessment and grading evaluation—types of and approaches to assessment and evaluation. Baylor University Academy for Teaching and Learning. **www.baylor.edu/atl/doc.php/306650.pdf**. Accessed May 9, 2021.
22. Boyle JA, Jenkins ZN, Franz TT, et al. Evaluation of student perceptions of introductory pharmacy practice experiences. *Curr Pharm Teach Learn*. 2020;12(6):633-640. doi:10.1016/j.cptl.2020.01.029.
23. Medina MS, Plaza CM, Stowe CD, et al. Center for the Advancement of Pharmacy Education 2013 Educational Outcomes. *Am J Pharm Educ*. 2013;77(8):162. doi: 10.5688/ajpe778162.
24. Haines ST, Pittenger AL, Stolte SK, et al. Core entrustable professional activities for new pharmacy graduates. *Am J Pharm Educ*. 2017;81(1):S2. doi: 10.5688/ajpe811S2.
25. Louiselle K, Elson EC, Oschman A, Duehlmeyer S. Impact of COVID-19 pandemic on pharmacy learners and preceptors. *Am J Health Syst Pharm*. 2020; 77(14): 1097-1098. doi: 10.1093/ajhp/zxaa127.
26. Watson S, Fuller K. Unanticipated learning opportunities for pharmacy students during COVID-19. *Pharmacy Times*, 2020. Podcast. **https://www.pharmacytimes.com/news/unanticipated-learning-opportunities-for-pharmacy-students-during-covid-19**. Accessed May 18, 2021.
27. Duty-Hour Requirements for Pharmacy Residencies. American Society of Health-System Pharmacists, 2015. **https://www.ashp.org/-/media/assets/professional-development/residencies/docs/duty-hour-requirements.ashx**. Accessed May 18, 2021.

CHAPTER 17
Care Flow Models with Integration of Learners into Telehealth Pharmacy Practice

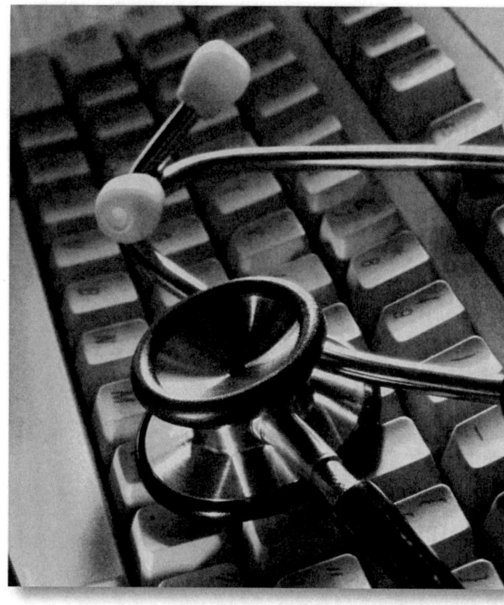

In the same way that IPPE, APPE, and residency clinical experiences can vary, rotations that incorporate telehealth pharmacy practice in full or in portions may also vary. Differences in care flow models for learning experiences include site setting, length of experience, type of learner(s), and option of remote care provided. The care flow model should also identify the points of learner contact and include a plan for transitions between live, telehealth, and/or hybrid models. For reference, a variety of Care Flow Model examples are included below.

VIDEO/TELEPHONIC EXAMPLES

Ambulatory Care IPPE Experience Layered with an APPE Student

The second pharmacy year ambulatory care IPPE experience met daily from 8–10:45 am. Students were prepared and precepted to engage in a pharmacy-run Diabetes Self-Management Education and Support (DSMES) service for a federally qualified health center (FQHC).

Structure

The ambulatory pharmacy practice site converted from providing live DSMES to providing services via telephone during the COVID-19 pandemic. Due to the confined space at the ambulatory site, learners transitioned from the clinic to meeting at the College of Pharmacy in order to meet social distancing guidelines. The preceptor had remote access to the clinic's electronic health record (EHR) and was provided a password-protected laptop for off-site use.

The clinic support staff scheduled 30-minute patient appointments (available times: 8:30 am–9:00 am; 9:30 am–10:00 am) for the diabetes education class. Patients usually had weekly 30-minute appointments for a total of four sessions. Thirty minutes were allowed between the end and beginning of patient appointments for student feedback and prep-work for the next patient. Second-year IPPE students were grouped into four students per day. Each group of IPPE students provided education to two patients per group.

Orientation and Student Preparation

Learners were provided the syllabus, clinical guidelines, patient education modules, expectations of professionalism, dress, and resources to review before the experience. Students were instructed to bring their laptops in order to access the materials during the experience.

Orientation to IPPE students was provided at 8:00 am on the first day to review the online prepping materials provided and to establish and evaluate baseline knowledge.

DOI 10.37573/9781585286928.017

The preceptor briefed the IPPE students on the evaluation methods that would be employed as well as the roles of the ambulatory pharmacist and APPE student. Expectations of professionalism were reiterated, as were due dates for self-directed learning. Students signed confidentiality agreements and the preceptor collected.

Before each patient session, the students were prepared to provide a quick medication reconciliation. The patient education module to be covered was reviewed with students. The preceptor or APPE student modeled communication strategies. Each of the four students was given responsibility for a section of the patient education module to discuss with the patient.

Student Debriefing

Following the patient visit, the preceptor debriefed students and assessed learner feedback and concerns.

The preceptor posed the following debriefing questions to the group:

"What did you think you did well?"

"In what areas could you improve on (list a specific event or tactic), or do you need more practice?"

"How did counseling via the telephone differ from in-person?"

"What patient care barriers may have been present today?"

"How did we ensure patient inclusivity and cultural sensitivity? Was this harder or easier via telephone?"

"What items would you want to convey to the patient's provider?"

Supplemental Activities

In addition to the two mornings of telehealth patient encounters, a self-directed case study DSMES SOAP note was required to supplement the experience. In the event of patient no-shows or gaps in the schedule, alternate activities were available, including developing a SOAP note on the patient that would have been seen, providing glucometer and point-of-care technique education, discussing practice guidelines, and reflecting on patient barriers to care.

IPPE/APPE Layered Learning

A layered learning experience was provided with Pharmacy Year 2 (PY2) IPPE students and an APPE academic or ambulatory monthly rotation student. The APPE student was provided access to the online class materials for the IPPE experience and was oriented to the ambulatory site, as well as to the structure of the IPPE experience.

In addition to their ambulatory care learning experience, the APPE student layered-learning responsibilities included involvement in precepting the IPPE students. The APPE student learning activities included writing up patients, gathering supplies, preparing students on the patient education modules, modeling communication strategies, and reviewing IPPE student SOAP notes. The APPE student also assisted the preceptor in real-time formative evaluations of students and providing feedback. The preceptor modeled the patient care activities and IPPE activities initially, allowing the APPE student to grow until the student's entrustability reached independent precepting.

AMBULATORY CARE APPE ROTATION EXAMPLE: BLOCK EXPERIENCE

Fourth-year experiential pharmacy students completed a remote ambulatory care APPE experience over a six-week period. This rotation took place in an outpatient clinic from 8:00 am–5:00 pm. Students were prepared to participate in the management of chronic disease state management, with specific focus on anticoagulation, diabetes, hypertension, hyperlipidemia, and smoking cessation.

Structure

The ambulatory pharmacy practice site was converted from a fully live in-clinic rotation to students completing patient care services via telephone and video-conferencing software remotely. The students, residents, and preceptors had remote access to the clinic's EHR.

Daily workflow was divided into three major parts: morning check-in meeting, lunch meeting, and end of the day check-out. The morning check-in meeting consisted of dedicated time with the preceptor and student(s) to discuss the plan for the day. This meeting was conducted over video-conference technology. The discussion included setting out expectations for the day, assigning students to specific patients to work up for anticoagulation management, diabetes management, hypertension management, and hyperlipidemia management, and also assigning students specific patients to complete medication reviews. Student(s) would then spend the morning completing these assigned tasks from home, as they had access to the electronic health records using home laptops and computers. Throughout the morning, students had the ability to contact the preceptor through telephone calls and video-conferencing with questions or concerns.

After the morning tasks were completed, the preceptor and student(s) would complete a lunch meeting, and the lunch meeting was completed over video-conference software, in the same manner as the morning check-in was conducted. During this dedicated time, student(s) would present patients from their morning workup. A tentative care plan was developed for each patient with preceptor guidance. The preceptor would then designate students to specific patients to complete the encounter. These encounters happened over the phone, as well as over video-conference, depending on the patient's preference or technological abilities. The preceptor was available at all times for questions or concerns brought up by the student or the patient. The software used gave the preceptor the ability to three-way into telephone calls or to enter the virtual patient encounter room through video-conferencing to monitor student progress, as well as to step in as needed for patient care. In addition, during the lunch meetings, the students would rotate each day, presenting on a 10-minute clinical pearl. The focus of these pearls was to teach their peer students and preceptor something unusual they has uncovered while working up patients the previous day that required searching through the literature for more information.

The last portion of the day concluded with an end-of-the-day check-out. Depending on patient load and clinical activities completed throughout the afternoon, this check-out was conducted as either a meeting or an email summarizing the afternoon's learning activities. Due to limited patient care access, some days required more longitudinal projects and did not always call for a meeting at the end of the day. If students were completing patient care activities, a meeting was held. Some examples of longitudinal projects that were completed by the students were clinical pearl preparation, research/quality improvement projects, medication-use evaluations, drug information questions, and topic discussion preparation. Students also helped create counseling sheets for patients to take home or to be shared via video-conferencing software for education regarding home monitoring of blood glucose and blood pressure, as well as strategies to start a diabetes-friendly diet and how to use a wide variety of injectable medications. Finally, depending on the time of year, students helped develop patient cases based on the real-life patients they were encountering via telehealth and assessment questions for underclassmen.

Orientation and Student Preparation

On the first day of the rotation, students were provided the syllabus, and expectations were reviewed. Students were oriented to the EHR and video-conferencing software, as well as how to access remote clinical resources. Baseline clinical knowledge was determined, and goals were set for each student.

Student Debriefing

As daily workflow was divided into three major parts, students had the opportunity to ask questions at each of the designated meeting times, and at the same time preceptors provided students feedback. This formative feedback was in addition to formal feedback given at the halfway mark and at the end of the rotation experience.

Longitudinal Ambulatory Care Resident Rotation, Example 1

As part of a PGY1 community pharmacy resident and PGY2 ambulatory care residency, residents would staff a hospital-based anticoagulation clinic one day every other week. This longitudinal rotation took place every other Friday morning from 8:00 am to 12:00 pm (or until the last patient was seen). Residents were prepared to participate in anticoagulation management for low health literacy and low-income patient population.

Structure

The rotation originated as a fully in-person clinic and was transitioned to a fully telephonic clinic. The general patient population consisted of low health literacy and limited access to transportation and healthcare. Patients were scheduled from 8:00 am to 12:00 pm in 30-minute increments. Each time slot had a maximum of five patients scheduled. For example, at 8:00 am, a maximum of five patients would be scheduled, and at 8:30 am an additional five patients. Due to barriers to care and to ensure that patients had a consistent way of obtaining an INR, patients presented to the clinic at the designated appointment time in order to have point-of-care or venous INR completed. The lead pharmacist then assigned each resident a specific timeframe to contact patients. For example, one resident would cover from 8:00 am–9:00 am, contacting a maximum of 10 patients. Pharmacy residents had the responsibility to work up patients, call and interview the patient, and develop a plan with follow-up. A hematologist was present onsite to help manage acute complications related to anticoagulation therapy. To reduce the potential for missed calls or lack of communication for critical INR, the in-clinic provider saw any patients with resulting INR <1.5 or >6.

Orientation and Resident Preparation

On the first day of the longitudinal rotation, residents were provided a syllabus and expectations were reviewed. Residents were oriented to the EHR and were given access to both the EHR and remote clinical resources. In addition to the syllabus, the residents were also provided with the clinic's specific procedures and an "anticoagulation guide" to review prior to seeing and/or communicating with patients.

Resident Debriefing

As this was a longitudinal rotation, residents received formative feedback throughout each shift covered. In addition, formal feedback was provided on a quarterly basis.

AMBULATORY CARE APPE ROTATION EXAMPLE: LONGITUDINAL EXPERIENCE

In a required ambulatory experience for the PGY1 pharmacy practice residency program, learners transitioned to working 100% offsite from the clinic setting. This initial transition allowed the PGY1 residents to meet the increased demands for inpatient staffing during the COVID-19 pandemic and paved the way for an innovative and efficient use of resident time and experience.

Structure

A typical day of the rotation was broken into morning and afternoon. Most morning sessions began at 7:30 am with residents remotely reviewing the scheduled patient visits for the day. The PGY1 residents also conducted telephonic interviews for scheduled patient visits to collect patient-specific subjective information that would be shared with the preceptor. These visits focused on the chronic disease states of anticoagulation, hypertension, and diabetes management. Once patients presented to the clinic, they were seen by the pharmacist preceptor to obtain objective information such as vitals and any pertinent labs. The PGY1 pharmacy resident and preceptor then met together via instant messaging, phone, or video-conferencing to discuss the pharmacotherapeutic plan. The plan was then provided to the patient live by the preceptor, or HIPAA-compliant video-conferencing was utilized for the resident learner to present.

The afternoon session began soon after the common lunch hour, which also served as the time for administrative meetings, preceptor feedback, journal clubs, site in-services, patient case presentations, and the like. During the afternoon, the PGY1 pharmacy resident followed up on lab results, coordinated with other providers and specialties, and performed any other duties for the morning's patients.

Orientation and Resident Preparation

As is normally the case for the experience, the resident was oriented with preceptor and site responsibilities and expectations and was given an overview of the learning experience, together with a shared calendar of activities. The provided resources also included are described in Tool for Essential Resources Required for Learner Experience in Chapter 16.

Resident Debriefing

The day concluded with an end-of-day check-out to discuss the lessons learned from the day, as well as any follow-up items and plan for the next day.

HYBRID EXAMPLES

Longitudinal PGY1 Ambulatory Care Rotation/Ambulatory Care APPE Rotation: Example

As part of a PGY1 residency, residents participated in a longitudinal rotation that took place weekly from 8:00 am to 5:00 pm. Learners (both students and residents) were prepared to participate in the management of chronic disease state management, with specific focus on anticoagulation, diabetes, hypertension, osteoporosis, and smoking cessation. However, the needs of the physicians were met as patients were referred to the pharmacy service.

Structure

This rotation originated as a fully in-person clinic and was transitioned to a hybrid clinic setting. As a layered-learning model, preceptors and residents were stationed in the clinic, while student(s) were stationed from home. Patients were able to complete encounters via telehealth or in person based on the patient's preference. As preceptors and residents were stationed in the clinic, they were responsible for seeing patients that presented to the clinic. However, in certain instances students were able to complete these encounters via video-conferencing software. For example, the student stationed from home, using video-conferencing software, would be brought up on a laptop in the exam room. The student would then proceed to interview the patient, who was present in clinic. Once the interview was completed, the resident or preceptor would take the laptop from the room to discuss the care plan for the patient. The student and resident or preceptor then presented the care plan to the patient.

In addition, residents were also responsible for delegating both patient care activities and longitudinal projects to students. As residents were seeing patients in the clinic, students were assigned to specific patients to work up for anticoagulation, diabetes, hypertension, hyperlipidemia, and osteoporosis management or smoking cessation assistance. The patients that students were responsible for were seen over video-conference or over the phone based on patient preference. Prior to each telehealth pharmacy practice appointment, students would meet with the preceptor to discuss patient workup and create a tentative plan for the patient.

Orientation and Learner Preparation

At the beginning of residency, residents were provided with a syllabus and expectations were reviewed. Baseline clinic knowledge was determined and goals were set. Residents were responsible for precepting APPE students after the first rotation block was completed with preceptor guidance. At the beginning of each APPE rotation block, students were provided with the syllabus, and expectations were reviewed in a similar manner to the resident's first day. For all learners, the EHR and software used for video conferences was reviewed, and each was provided access to the EHR at home, as well as remote clinical resources.

Learner Debriefing

For student learners, the preceptor and residents were available at all times during the telehealth encounter for questions or concerns brought up by the student or the patient. The software used provided the preceptor the ability to three-way into telephone calls or enter the virtual patient encounter room through video-conferencing to monitor student progress, as well as step in as needed for patient care. Formative feedback was provided to students after each patient encounter, and formal feedback was provided at both the midpoint of the rotation and the end of the rotation.

For resident learners, the preceptor was available at all times. However, more independence was given to the resident as the longitudinal rotation progressed. Formative feedback was provided as needed, and formal feedback was provided on a quarterly basis.

BARRIERS WITH SUGGESTED SOLUTIONS ASSOCIATED WITH CARE FLOW MODELS

Barrier 1: Technology Difficulties

- Innate issues with technology can be a problem for learners, preceptors, and patients alike. Learners may not have the appropriate technology/hardware to be able to run specific telehealth software or the electronic health record. This situation can be further complicated if Internet connection is unstable or nonexistent.
- For learners without appropriate resources at their home (such as reliable Internet or a computer) additional accommodations may be required and will be dependent on the available resources of that site. If there are unused meeting spaces at the site, the learner may be able to be onsite in these nonpatient care areas in order to obtain Wifi Internet access through the institution while following appropriate physical distancing recommendations. Further, if they are onsite, it may be possible for the learner to utilize computers, tablets, and/or telephones owned by the institution in order to deliver the patient care services. This may be preferred by the institution to ensure the devices utilized are appropriately encrypted and protected to prevent the unauthorized spread of patient health information (PHI) inadvertently. Additionally, this will ensure that the software required will be available to the learner and be consistent with the software programs available and utilized by the institution, the precepting pharmacist, and the patient.
- Telephonic services provided by learners at their house—Jabber, Google Voice, *67 (although "no show" rates may increase if a blocked number is displayed on the patient's call waiting) instead of using their personal phone number.

Solution 1: Advance Preparation for Technology Difficulties with Prespecified Protocol

- Technology issues are inevitable and to a degree unavoidable. As part of rotation preparation, preceptors should develop a handout or flowsheet to help mitigate some of the avoidable issues associated with technology issues, as well as learn what to do if an inevitable technology issue occurs. For example, a handout to mitigate avoidable issues would consist of keeping technology and software up-to-date, completing training associated with software, available troubleshooting contact information for specific software, and so on. If technology issues arise, a flowsheet would consist of steps to take if the Internet connection is unstable or goes out.

Barrier 2: Counseling Can Be Challenging for Administration/ Hands-On Activities

- Patient education for telehealth comes with its own challenges. A major portion of a learner's job in an ambulatory care setting is to educate patients on the medications they are taking, including proper administration. One of the most common ways pharmacists educate patients is through the teach-back method. Via telehealth, the teach-back method can be completed for general counseling information, but it can be challenging to complete for proper administration of nonoral medications. This creates challenges for pharmacist preceptors and learners to come up with creative ways to overcome.

Solution 2: Early Preparation to Optimize Communication

- There are a variety of ways barriers associated with counseling can be overcome. For example, learners and preceptors can use screen sharing with administration videos when a sample drug or device is not available. It also may be beneficial to email instructions to a patient instead of relying on an after-visit summary to print. Learners can help set patients up with online health records so that it will be easier to communicate with their healthcare providers if they have questions after the appointment is completed. In addition, learners and preceptors can call the pharmacy where the patient will pick up their new medication and further discuss with the pharmacist to help with counseling.

Pharmacy practice and, in turn, pharmacy education will continue to expand and evolve as the needs of both learners and patients change. To meet current and future needs, telehealth rotations and learning experiences have been developed and have barely tapped potential benefits for learners. As previously stated, ACPE and ACCP do not give specific recommendations or requirements for creating or transitioning to telehealth rotations.[1] The wide variety of "tools" presented throughout this section can be used to create innovative rotational experiences for students and residents, which will not only improve their learning and development, but also result in better patient care.

Preceptors, student pharmacists, and residents would be well served to embrace the telehealth platform. Market analyses and patient feedback all suggest that telehealth is not only increasingly popular, but increasingly expected within healthcare. As the *Harvard Business Review* forecasts, "In a few years, the idea of receiving medical treatment exclusively at a doctor's office or hospital will seem quaint. . . . by coordinating care more effectively and offering daily support—through mobile communication and remote monitoring—along with community outreach, companies can help shift care to more timely, home-based, and less costly interventions . . . in the next decade, these trends will create a veritable gold rush in patient data and consumer options."[2]

REFERENCES

1. Accreditation Council for Pharmacy Education. Guidance memos from ACPE to schools. **https://www.acpe-accredit.org/wp-content/uploads/guidance-memos-from-ACPE-to-the-schools-consolidated-5-8-20.pdf**. Accessed May 5, 2021.
2. Subramanian S, Dumont C, Dankert C, Wong A. Personalized technology will upend the doctor-patient relationship. *Harvard Business Review*, June 30, 2015. **hbr.org/2015/06/personalized-technology-will-upend-the-doctor-patient-relationship#**. May 18, 2021.

SECTION 5: CLINICAL VIGNETTE

Scenario

Because of a recent public health emergency, your clinic wants to limit the number of individuals onsite. You are going to start providing services remotely. You have an advanced pharmacy practice experience (APPE) student who is to start with you next week. You have no idea how long you will need to work remotely. What are some important questions that you need to consider as you are trying to design a remote learning experience for your learner?

Response

One of the first items you should evaluate is whether your learner will be able to access the electronic health record from home. Ensure that your organizational/clinic policies allow learners to remotely access patient information and that the infrastructure allows nonclinic devices to connect to the electronic health record. A next step would be to determine if there is a platform that allows for three-way calling or group video visits so that you can include your learner on your CCM calls. You will want to ensure that expectations on a remote learning experience are clear, including applying HIPAA-regulations at home. You may even consider adapting your current APPE syllabus to account for remote experiences.

A more detailed list of considerations can be found in the "Site Preparation Checklist."

INDEX

Page numbers followed by b refer to boxes, f to figures, and t to tables.

N

O

P

U

V

W

Z

FSC
www.fsc.org
MIX
Papier | Fördert gute Waldnutzung
FSC® C083411

Kolibri 360 GmbH
Ferdinand-Jühlke-Straße 7
99095 Erfurt, Deutschland
produktsicherheit@kolibri360.de